ADVANCED DENTAL HISTOLOGY

A DENTAL PRACTITIONER HANDBOOK
SERIES EDITED BY DONALD D. DERRICK DDS, LDS RCS

ADVANCED DENTAL HISTOLOGY

J. W. OSBORN
PHD, BDS(LOND), FDS RCS(ENG)

*Professor and Chairman,
Department of Oral Biology,
Faculty of Dentistry,
The University of Alberta
Edmonton, Alberta, Canada*

and

A. R. TEN CATE
BDS, BSC, PHD (LOND)

*Dean of the Faculty of Dentistry
University of Toronto
Ontario, Canada*

Fourth Edition

WRIGHT · PSG
BRISTOL . LONDON . BOSTON
1983

© **John Wright & Sons Ltd**, 1983

All Rights Reserved. No part of this publication may be reproduced, stored in a retrieval system, or transmitted in any form or by any means, electronic, mechanical, photocopying, recording or otherwise, without the prior permission of the Copyright owner.

Published by
John Wright & Sons Ltd, 823–825 Bath Road, Bristol BS4 5NU, England.
John Wright PSG Inc., 545 Great Road, Littleton, Massachusetts 01460, USA.

First edition, 1967
Second edition, 1971
Third edition, 1976
Fourth edition, 1983

British Library Cataloguing in Publication Data
Osborn, J. W.
    Advanced dental histology.—4th ed.
    ——. (A Dental practitioner handbook)
    1. Teeth   2. Histology
    I. Title   II. Ten Cate, A. R. III. Series
    611'. 0189' 314   RK307

ISBN 0 7236 0671 4

Library of Congress Catalog Card Number: 82–62618

Typeset and Printed in Great Britain by
John Wright & Sons (Printing) Ltd at The Stonebridge Press, Bristol BS4 5NU.

PREFACE

Recently each of us has separately been involved in the publication of undergraduate texts covering more or less the whole of dental anatomy, as opposed to the limited but more advanced dental histology reviewed here. We still feel that the material contained in this book is suited to undergraduates despite the fact that much of it does not appear in our other texts. This small book allows us to focus in depth on the teeth themselves, an exercise that would tend to unbalance a text covering the whole of dental anatomy.

Once again we have rewritten most of the chapters, not only in the addition of new material and the deletion of old—six years is a long time—but also because there always seems to be a better way of arranging current facts and hypotheses. If we started a new edition today it would probably be quite different from this one!

J. W. O.
A. R. T. C.

PREFACE TO THE FIRST EDITION

This book is not intended to be an orthodox textbook of dental histology but rather a supplement dealing with the latest, and often most controversial, aspects of the subject. Nor is it claimed that this book is fully comprehensive.

The rapid advances made in recent years in the field of dental histology involve the application of new disciplines, the results of which are to be found in an ever increasing range of scientific periodicals. In consequence, it has become increasingly difficult for students to find the time, and indeed the facilities, to collate this information from perusal of the original literature. Furthermore, the time lapse between completion of a manuscript and the appearance of a book is such as to preclude the incorporation of the latest information on any subject. It seemed to the authors, therefore, a worth while service to review these latest advances, and to present them in a series of short essays in the least dogmatic manner. They are based upon the dental histology portion of the pre-clinical course given to students of dentistry at Guy's Hospital. Many of the ideas presented herein are still in the formative stage and may or may not come to fruition in the future. Nevertheless, they are included in the hope of providing a stimulus for further study and enquiry on the part of the reader.

If the rapid advances in this subject over the past few years continue in the future, it is anticipated that this book will require frequent revision if it is to be of continuing value. Realizing this, the book has been written so as to facilitate rapid revision by virtue of its simplified line diagrams and absence of photographic plates.

Every effort has been made to produce an authoritative book at low cost, consistent with the policy of constant revision. Rather than burden the reader with a long list of references to each chapter, only those which are readily available in most libraries are quoted, from which further specific references can be obtained.

February, 1967

W.A.G.
J.W.O.
A.R.T.C.

CONTENTS

1. The Investigation of Tissues — 1
2. The Cell — 12
3. The Tooth in situ — 25
4. The Role of Ectomesenchyme in Tooth Formation and Induction — 28
5. The Early Development of the Teeth — 35
6. Morphogenesis — 46
7. Growth of the Tooth Germ — 56
8. The Blood Supply to the Teeth — 63
9. Collagen — 69
10. Hard Tissue Genesis — 75
11. Bone — 89
12. Dentinogenesis — 94
13. The Dentine Pulp Complex — 104
14. Dentine Sensitivity — 109
15. Amelogenesis — 118
16. Enamel Structure — 137
17. Cementogenesis and Cement Structure — 150
18. Root Formation — 156
19. The Periodontium — 161
20. Physiological Tooth Movement — 171
21. The Dento-gingival Junction — 183
22. The Final Investments of the Crown of the Tooth — 193
23. Age Changes in the Dental Tissues — 198
    Index — 205

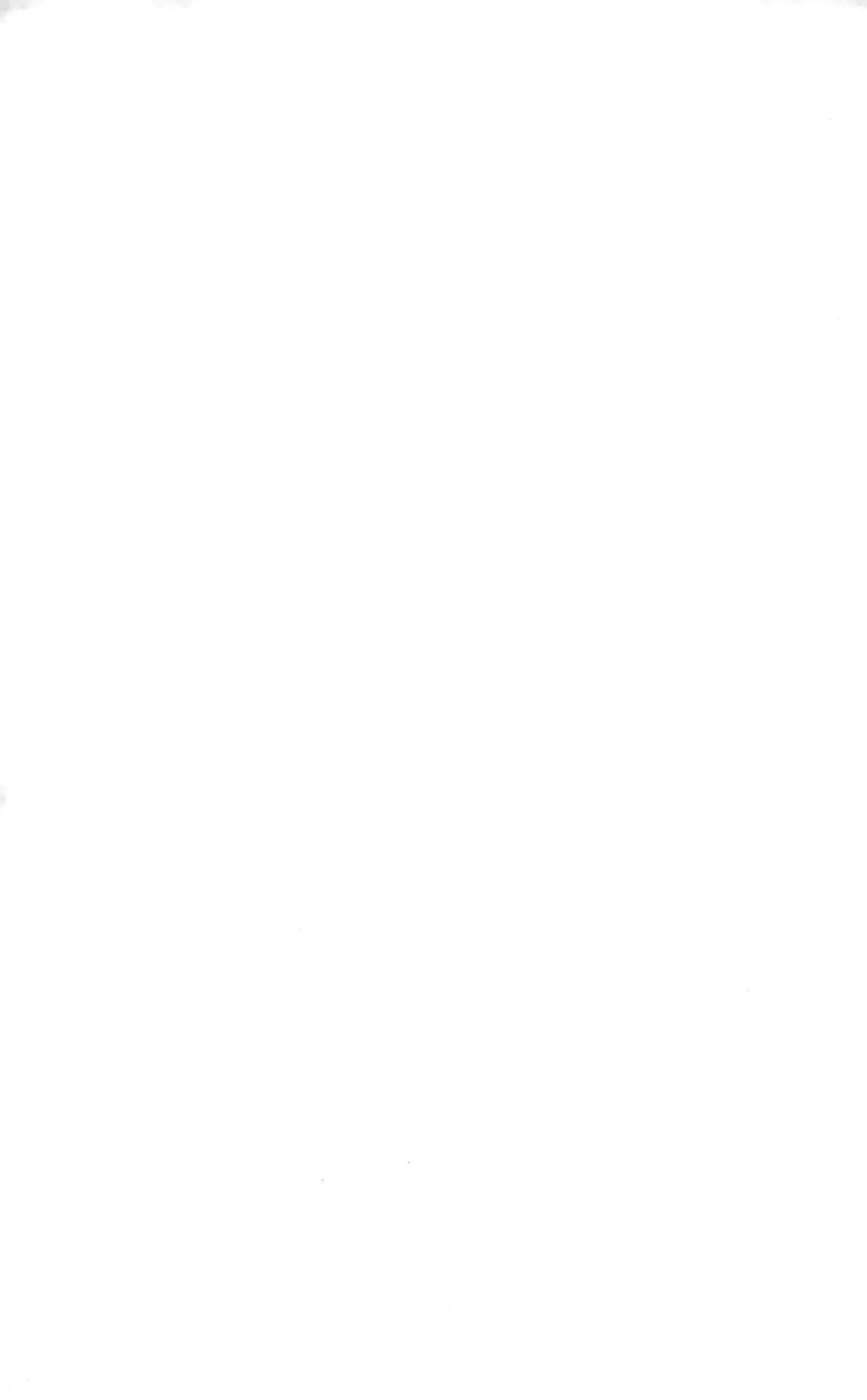

CHAPTER 1

THE INVESTIGATION OF TISSUES

The aim of the chapter is to give an outline of the more important methods which are used to determine the structure and function of the dental tissues and to indicate a few of their limitations.

LIGHT MICROSCOPY

By far the most common tool used in the investigation of tissues is the light microscope, which in general requires the preparation of sections thin enough to transmit light. The preparation of thin sections of dental tissues necessitates either demineralization of hard tissues with the loss of the highly mineralized enamel or, if demineralization is to be avoided, the grinding of slices of dental tissue with the consequent loss of the soft tissue elements.

A wide variety of chemicals has been used to stain demineralized sections in order to make the thin, and therefore largely transparent, material visible under the light microscope. It is obvious that these stained sections appeared very different prior to being pickled (fixed), dehydrated and wax-embedded, and yet most of our knowledge of the histological structure of the body and much of our knowledge of how the body functions, has been learned by studying these stained remnants of the original tissue. The confidence with which interpretations are made is based on what is known as the 'reproducible artefact'.

It is of little value to mix together a number of chemicals and after staining a section with them to describe the appearance of the tissue in that section. The proportions and concentrations of the materials and the time of staining must be carefully measured and controlled. The effect of using different proportions, concentrations and staining times is studied and finally the combination which produces the best staining of tissue is selected. This type of experimenting is fundamental to light microscopy and many of the well-known staining procedures are named after the persons who originally formulated them (e.g. Mallory, van Gieson, Masson).

If a new tissue is to be studied, one or more of the well-known staining procedures is chosen on the basis of the components of the tissues which are selectively stained by the method. The effects of the staining procedure are studied on a large number of sections until it is verified that the stain regularly produces the same picture; in other words that the 'artefact is reproducible'.

Frequently we are interested in the overall appearance of a tissue rather than the minutiae of a single component contained within the tissue. One of the standard combinations of stains used for general histology is that of haematoxylin and eosin. Mature haematoxylin is a basic stain and therefore attaches to acidic materials (e.g. the DNA and RNA of cells). Therefore nuclei are stained blue and cells rapidly synthesizing material (cells with a high proportion of RNA in the cytoplasm) will have a blueish cytoplasm. Eosin has an affinity for most materials and will stain all components red. It is therefore referred to as a 'counterstain'. Without this counterstain the material not stained by haematoxylin would be colourless and largely invisible.

For a more detailed study of some of the components of a tissue more selective staining procedures are required. Indeed, the value of a stain frequently depends on the specificity with which it will react with a component of a tissue. For example, certain silver solutions will precipitate on nerve fibres but at the same time are also bound by other materials in sections (*see* Chapter 12) which mimic fibres. Although this staining is reproducible the value of sections stained in this way is often limited because of the difficulty in distinguishing which component of the tissue has been affected. Therefore, in the use of silver stains elaborate methods have been introduced in attempts to confine the precipitate to one specific component of the tissue.

Some of the most specific of staining techniques are those used in histochemistry. Histochemical techniques attempt to demonstrate microscopically the chemistry of cells and tissues. Such techniques usually depend on specific chemical reactions which form a coloured reaction product visible with the light microscope. An example illustrating the principles of histochemical practice is the simultaneous coupling azo-dye method for demonstrating the location of the enzyme acid phosphatase in tissue sections. The term 'acid phosphatase' is applied to the organic catalyst which, operating at an acid pH, splits phosphates from organic esters. Sections must be prepared without inactivating the enzyme or dislocating it from its intracellular position. In the case of the dental tissues this normally implies the cutting of unfixed, undemineralized frozen sections in order not to denature the enzyme. To such sections a solution is applied which is buffered at an acid pH (the working pH of the enzyme) and contains a substrate (sodium α-naphthyl phosphate) which the enzyme can split, together with a relatively colourless azo-dye. The enzyme splits the phosphate from the substrate exposing the naphthyl group which instantly combines with the azo-dye to produce a coloured reaction product at the site of the enzyme activity (*Fig. 1.1*). Using this method it is possible to demonstrate the activity of acid phosphatase in a wide variety of tissues.

It is sometimes helpful to view sections unstained. This is particularly true of the ground sections so commonly used in the study of dental

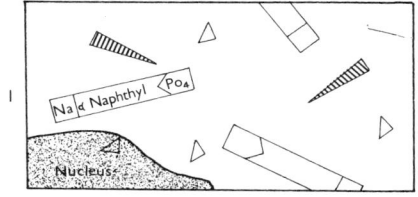

Diagrammatic appearance of section containing enzymes (cross-hatched) and nucleus (stippled). The section has been treated with sodium α-naphthyl phosphate and azo-dye (triangle) in a buffered medium.

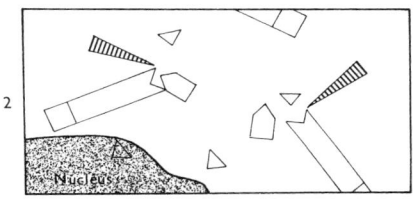

The enzyme splits off the PO_4^{2+} and the sodium α-naphthyl component competes for the azo-dye.

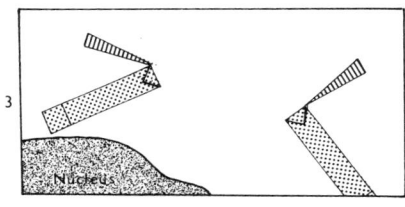

The PO_4^{2+} is replaced by the azo-dye to produce a coloured reaction product at the sites of enzyme activity.

Fig. 1.1. Diagrams of the steps in the simultaneous coupling azo-dye method for demonstrating the location of the enzyme acid phosphatase in tissue section.

tissues. In this case the picture seen under the microscope is produced due to differences between the light absorption, refractive indices and optical interference of the component tissues. For instance, the dentinal tubules in a ground section are seen due to the difference of refractive index between the air contained in the tubule and that of the intertubular dentine. If the tubule becomes filled with calcified material, the tubule then has a similar refractive index to the intertubular material and the dentine becomes transparent. Probably the borders of enamel prisms are seen under the light microscope because light is reflected at the boundary between the prism sheath (refractive index (R.I.) is that of protein and is 1·3) and the hydroxyapatite of the prisms (R.I. = 1·7). The striae of Retzius, a structural component of enamel, appear brown by transmitted light because in the region of the striae blue light (shorter wavelength) is scattered away from the direction of viewing.

Frequently the optical heterogeneity of a specimen is difficult or impossible to see using the normal optical system of the light microscope. Phase contrast, interference and polarization microscopy techniques use different optical systems to make these heterogeneities visible. For example, the phase contrast microscope identifies very small, otherwise invisible, changes in refractive index.

ELECTRON MICROSCOPY

Transmission Electron Microscopy (TEM)

The limit of resolution of the light microscope (the ability to distinguish two points as separate) is about 0·1 µm and is dependent upon the wavelength of light. Attempts have been made to improve resolution by utilizing radiations of shorter wavelengths, such as X-rays, but the difficulty here is the inability to focus X-rays; hence at present X-ray microscopy is not a practical proposition. Far greater success has been achieved, however, by the use of electron beams which, although not part of the electro-magnetic spectrum, can be produced with a much shorter wavelength than light radiation. Also, as electrons are electrically charged, they can readily be focused by means of electro-magnets. The principles of electron microscopy are the same as for light microscopy (*Fig. 1.2*), except that electrons are used instead of light for illumination the specimen and electro-magnets are substituted for the glass lenses of the light microscope. Because of the short wavelength, the resolving power of the electron microscope is over 100 times greater than that of the light microscope and true magnifications of up to × 1 000 000 are possible. The preparation of any tissues for electron microscopy is complicated by the fact than extremely thin sections are necessary as electrons have little penetrative power, and this raises additional technical problems so far as the dental hard tissues are concerned.

Because the wavelengths of electron beams are outside the visible spectrum a black and white image of the tissue being examined is produced on a screen. Many cell organelles are bounded by lipids. These can be stained with the heavy metal in osmium tetroxide which absorbs electrons. On such electron micrographs the membranes appear dark (they have absorbed electrons).

While the electron microscope has many advantages over the light microscope, the preparation and study of sections are very much more difficult. Therefore, whereas the cells studied by the light microscopist may be numbered in thousands, only a few may be studied at any one time by the electron microscopist. This poor sampling rate limits the value of electron microscopy. Furthermore, for many years much of electron microscopy was merely descriptive. For instance, numerous types of vesicle were described—coated vesicles, granular vesicles, dense vesicles, light vesicles, dark vesicles and so on—without much knowledge of their function. It is only recently that sufficient knowledge of cell activity has been acquired to enable functions to be allotted to many of the structures

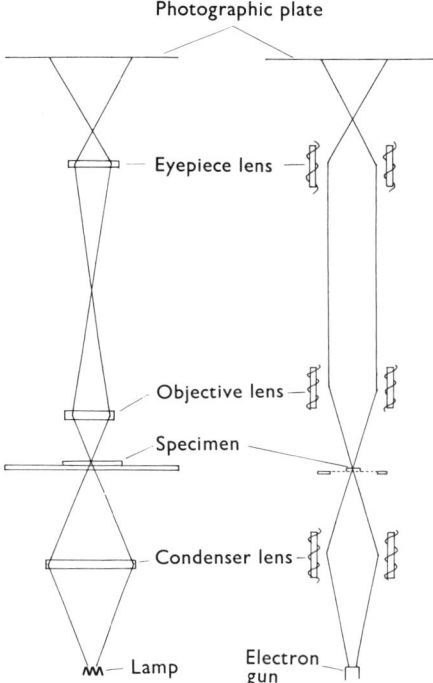

Fig. 1.2. Diagram illustrating the similar principles of light and electron microscopy.

seen in electron micrographs of cells. Recently histochemical and autoradiographic (*see below*) techniques have been used in electron microscopy and such techniques have made it possible to interpret the function of some of these organelles.

Scanning Electron Microscopy (SEM)

Both light and electron microscopes produce an image in two dimensions of what is substantially a two-dimensional slice of tissue. It is often difficult to visualize the appearance of the tissue in three dimensions.

In the scanning electron microscope a narrow beam of electrons is made to scan the surface of tissues which have been coated with a reflective metal, rather like the spot on a television screen. The scanning beam is reflected from the surface of the tissue and ultimately on to a viewing screen. Because the beam obeys the normal laws of reflection an apparently three dimensional image is produced of the surface scanned, based on the equivalent of light and shade. The image produced may be magnified up to 50 000 times.

Apart from the fact that scanning electron microscopy does not require the very demanding techniques of section cutting necessary for transmission electron microscopy (a surface is 'scanned' by electrons rather than electrons being transmitted through an ultra-thin section), the instrument has the advantage of providing an incredible depth of focus. With the light microscope at a magnification of about × 1000 (its limit of useful magnification) less than a 1 μm depth of section is in focus: if we want to examine the whole thickness of a 5 μm thick section we must rack the microscope up and down. But at the relatively enormous magnifications used in scanning electron microscopy, most of the irregularities of a surface being examined are in sharp focus. It is for this reason that the scanning electron microscope has been so valuable in studying, for example, the surfaces of teeth. But it must always be remembered that for most other tissues a coated surface is being examined. Failure to do so has led to some false interpretations.

HISTOLOGICAL MARKERS

In order to understand the dynamics of cells and the metabolism of tissues, markers are used to identify specific components. These can be either radioactive or immunological markers.

Radioactive Markers

Autoradiography uses radioactive markers. In this instance a radioactive atom such as calcium (^{42}Ca) or hydrogen (^3H) is substituted for its normal counterpart in a substance used by the body. For example ^3H (tritium) can be substituted into a nucleic acid such as thymidine (tritium-labelled or tritiated thymidine) or an amino-acid. Alternatively radioactive calcium or sulphur can be introduced into the body of an experimental animal. In all cases the radioactively labelled substance is (presumably) metabolized by the body in the same way as its normal counterpart. Subsequently, this material can be traced in tissue sections due to its radioactivity. For instance, radioactive proline can be injected into the peritoneum of a rat. The proline is absorbed, circulates in the bloodstream and becomes utilized in the formation of collagen in the periodontal ligament. Two days later the animal is killed and sections of the periodontal ligament are prepared by normal histological methods. The sections are now taken into a dark room and coated with a thin layer of photographic emulsion. After a few weeks in the dark room (the actual time depends on the half-life of the labelled atom) the emulsion is reduced over the spots where the radioactive proline is present. The emulsion is then developed photographically. When the stained section is viewed through the now transparent emulsion, the silver grains indicate the exact spots where the radioactive proline has been incorporated (*Fig. 1.3*). Following the initial injection of labelled proline we can kill animals at weekly intervals and expect, by autoradiography, to find evidence of the radioactive proline. When we no longer find evidence of it we can argue that all the newly formed collagen which incorporated the radioactive proline has now been removed. In other words we have an idea of how rapidly collagen is turned over in the periodontal ligament.

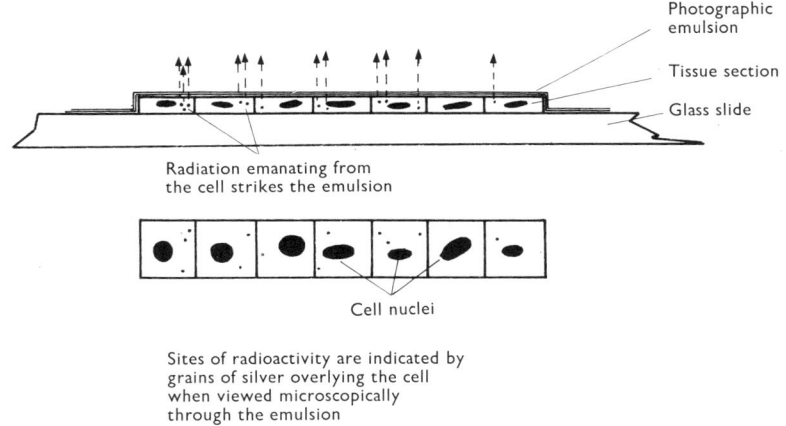

Fig. 1.3. Diagram illustrating the principle of autoradiography.

In one experiment the apices of continually growing rodent incisors were blocked with a filling material. Labelled calcium was now injected into the abdomens and a few weeks later the animals were killed. Ground sections of the incisors were cut and covered with photographic emulsion in a dark room. Subsequently it was observed that radioactive calcium had been incorporated in the newly formed enamel. Because the pulp cavity had previously been blocked, it is evident that the calcium must have come from the ameloblasts via the bloodstream proving that the enamel organ and not the pulp provided the mineral for enamel.

Immunological Markers

Techniques using immunological markers are becoming increasingly important because of the extreme specificity of antibodies. Suppose we are interested in the distribution of type IV collagen, basement membrane collagen, in tooth germs. A purified source of type IV collagen, usually the lens capsule of the eye or kidney glomerulus, is injected into rabbits (for example) where the production of antibodies is stimulated. When, usually following repeated injections of antigen (type IV collagen), the blood level of antibodies in the rabbit is sufficiently high, its serum is isolated and the required antibodies purified. Frozen sections of mouse tooth germ are now cut and the sections incubated in a solution of the antibody which, as is the nature of antibodies, binds to all substances containing the antigenic site (in this case a site on type IV collagen). The section is now incubated with an anti-antibody together with a dye, fluorescein, which binds to the anti-antibody. When the section is viewed by ultraviolet light it fluoresces in the places where the sandwich, fluorescein–anti-antibody–antibody, has attached to it thereby identifying the sites of type IV collagen. It will be appreciated that the technique is successful only if the antibody is specific for type IV collagen. If some other substance in the body contains the same antigenic site, it also will stain. The technique is modified for electron microscopy by using (electron-dense) ferritin as a marker instead of fluorescein.

BIOCHEMISTRY

Every protein has three levels of structure which can be analysed: the proportion of the amino-acids it contains, the order of these amino-acids in the protein chain and, lastly, the three-dimensional arrangement of the resulting chain or chains. Of these levels of structure the first (the proportion of the amino-acids) is the most easy to study and the third is extremely difficult and not often attempted.

It is not difficult to break the peptide bonds in a protein chain, thereby reducing the protein to its constituent amino-acids. In order to analyse the proportion of these amino-acids chromatographic techniques are used. Increasingly more sophisticated methods are being developed but the principle involved is the same. A mixture of substances is made to move through a network or filter which retards those substances that have, for example, a higher molecular weight or a positive charge. For instance, in column chromatography the sample to be analysed is washed through a long column of resinous material. The resinous material may be chosen preferentially to retard positively charged amino-acids and also have a pore size which will slow down the rate of movement of all the larger amino-acids. The amino-acids pass through the column at different rates (according to their size and charge) and can be collected separately at the bottom of the column (*Fig. 1.4*). Subsequently the proportions of each amino-acid can be determined. The data are usually given as numbers of amino-acids per 1000 residues. For instance, collagen in human dentine has 319 glycine molecules in every 1000 amino-acids, i.e. the collagen contains about one-third glycine.

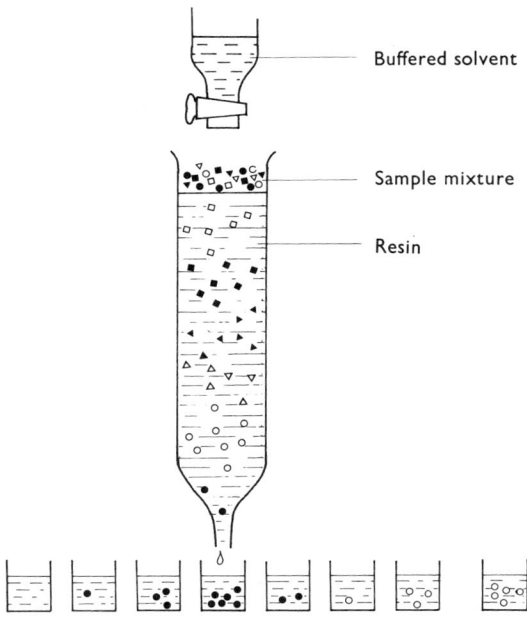

Fig. 1.4. The principle of column chromatography.

The sequence of amino-acids in a protein can be analysed by enzymatically chopping off successive terminal amino-acids from a pure preparation of the protein and at each step identifying the newly released amino-acid. By careful manual techniques about 10 amino-acids can be identified before the remaining mixture becomes too disrupted, but machines, amino-acid sequencers, can increase this to about 60 amino-acids. The major problem with this technique is the purification of the protein under study.

MICRORADIOGRAPHIC METHODS

X-rays have a common application in the study of dental tissues. Most readers will be familiar with the conventional radiographs used in diagnostic medicine. Such radiographs rely on the use of X-rays generated at high voltage and of short wavelength, the so-called 'hard' X-rays. The same principle is involved with contact microradiography. The specimen is placed in contact with a recording photographic emulsion and exposed to 'soft' X-rays, generated at low voltages and of longer wavelengths. The

X-rays are differentially absorbed by the specimen, depending on the number, the kind of atoms and their capacity to absorb X-rays. From the resulting photographic record information can be gained about the overall pattern, degree and detail of mineralization. For instance, peritubular dentine can easily be recognized using microradiography.

EXPERIMENTAL METHODS

Such methods usually depend upon altering the environment of the living tissue being studied in a specific way and observing any response with many of the techniques already described. Included in this category are experimental methods such as those designed to reveal the effect of specific dietary deficiencies and additions, ablation studies and tissue culture studies. There are many other techniques in this category which have been used to investigate the dental tissues. Examples will be referred to in later chapters.

CONTROLS

It is particularly important to use 'controls' in experimental work. Experiments, if they are to have any value, are almost always designed to test a hypothesis. In other words, the worker knows, or hopes he knows, the result he will obtain. Control experiments are designed to test the validity of the conclusions which might later be made from the results. Suppose we suspect, but do not know, that dentine contains nerves. Histological sections of dozens of teeth are prepared and stained in order to demonstrate nerve fibres. In one such series of studies in the 1930s the particular technique used seemed to show that every dentinal tubule contained nerve fibres. A control experiment could have taken the following form. In a group of animals, the inferior dental nerve would be cut and the animals killed 2 or 3 weeks later. All the sensory nerve fibres in the lower teeth would have degenerated. If histological sections of these teeth had been prepared, it would have been found that all the dentinal tubules still contained nerve fibres. The controls would have demonstrated that the stain was not picking out sensory nerve fibres of the inferior dental nerve, but probably staining the contents of dentinal tubules.

INTERPRETATION

Finally, there is always the problem of correctly interpreting data. The classic example in this field is an experiment in which fleas were taught to jump on a word of command. It was found that if either of the two front pairs of legs was removed, fleas continued to jump on the word of command, but they did not respond if their back legs were removed. Evidently amputation of the hind legs leads to deafness in fleas. This is not an outrageous parody of scientific interpretations. It is by no means improbable that similar mistakes are made in the interpretation of many experiments, particularly those analysing complex biochemical systems which often involve unknown intermediate reactions.

CHAPTER 2

THE CELL

It is difficult to understand how such complex structures as cells evolved, let alone multicellular organisms. An interesting suggestion is that some of the complexity of unicellular *eukaryotes* (cells containing organelles, such as amoeba, as opposed to *prokaryotes,* such as bacteria, which do not contain organelles) evolved symbiotically. For example, mitochondria-like organisms containing DNA invaded and lived in symbiosis with another organism, the host making use of the ATP generated by its invader, and the invader depending on the host for its raw materials. Finally, each became totally dependent on the other. This theory can account for the origin of the (extranuclear) DNA associated with (self-replicating) mitochondria. In a similar way cilia may have developed from a flagellated symbiote and, in the plant world, chloroplasts from an originally free-living invader.

Colonies can develop from aggregates of originally isolated unicellular organisms, resulting in an opportunity for advantageous specialization. Peripheral cells specialize in the collection of raw materials and central cells specialize in the processing of these materials. From such simple multicellular organisms, new types of cells evolved and contributed increasing complexity, each new type of cell being more specialized and efficient at its own particular function but being ever more dependent on the host.

The fact that all the different cell types in a multicellular organism develop from a single parent leads to a fundamental similarity between the cell types in an organism (*Fig. 2.1*).

PLASMA MEMBRANE

Electron microscopy is sometimes referred to as the study of membranes because these are the lipid-containing structures which are made electron-dense, and therefore visible in the microscope, by the adsorption of stains such as osmium used in the preparation of tissues.

The most important function of membranes is to isolate chemicals and thereby concentrate reactants and prevent other uncontrolled reactions. Some small molecular weight substances can pass through the membrane but the movement of most reactants is controlled by receptors, sited on or in the membranes, which respond to other chemical substances or the reactants themselves by opening or closing pores in the membrane. An open pore may allow chemicals to pass through by diffusion or by the

THE CELL

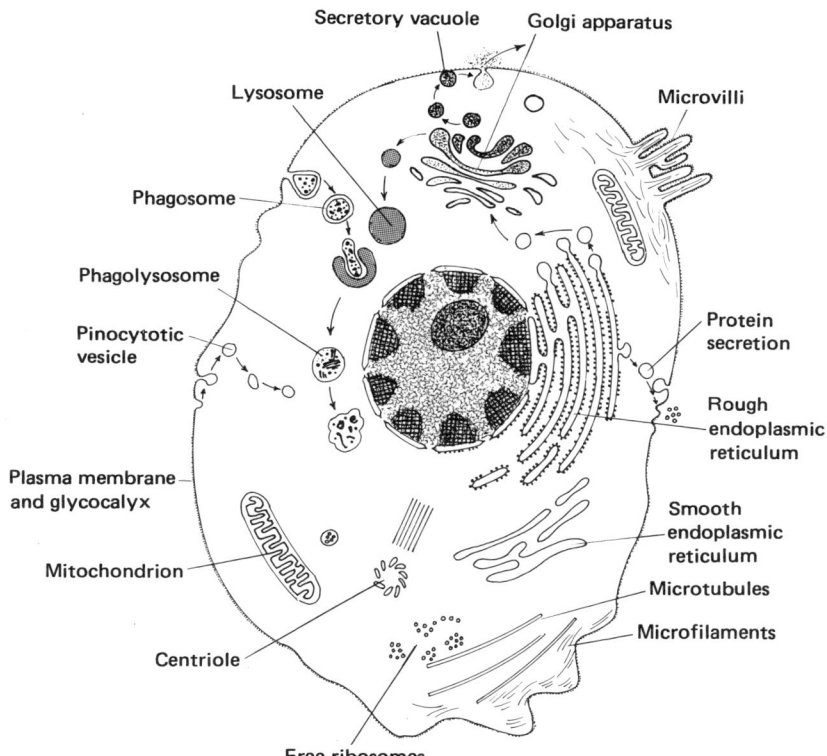

Fig. 2.1. Ultrastructure of organelles which may be found in a cell. (After Warwick R. and Williams P. L. (1980) in: *Gray's Anatomy*. Edinburgh Churchill Livingstone.)

action of a pump (active transport). The major structural features of a membrane are therefore the membrane itself, receptors, pores and pumps. All are constructed from organic molecules.

Structure

The cell is bounded by its plasma membrane outside which is a glycocalyx composed of glycoproteins. The glycocalyx may strengthen the plasma membrane, give the cell an electrostatic charge and filter substances thereby controlling cell activity.

The major part of the membrane consists of two layers (*Fig. 2.2*), an inner and outer phospholipid layer. The phospholipids have hydrophobic

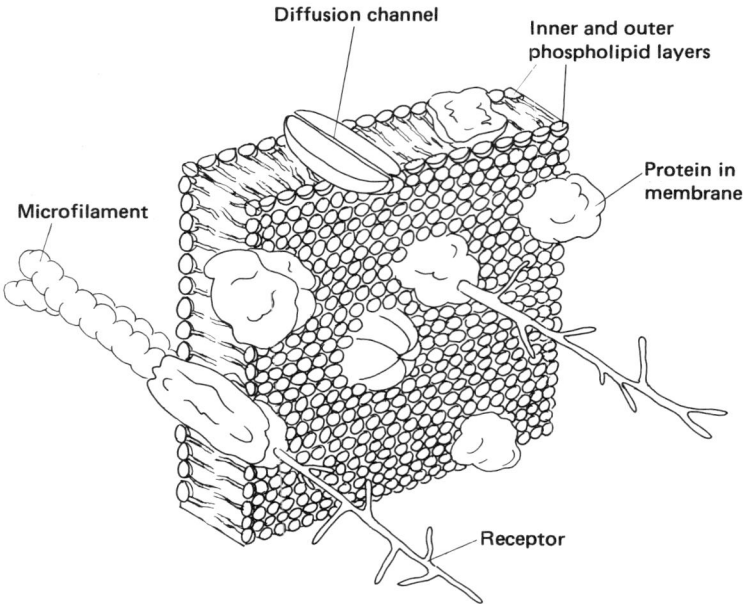

Fig. 2.2. The structure of plasma membrane (After Warwick R. and Williams P. L. in *Gray's Anatomy.*)

and hydrophilic ends. If the phospholipids are separated and mixed with water, they float on the surface with their hydrophobic ends out of the water thereby automatically aligning themselves. The phospholipid parts of the membrane could therefore be self-constructing with proteins later being incorporated.

The membrane is punctured by pores which are lined by proteins. The size of the pore is related to the (three-dimensional) conformation of its protein wall and this may be controlled by the environment and/or by enzymes also contained in or lying on the membrane.

Receptor molecules may either lie on the surface of the membrane or pass right through it, one end extending into the glycocalyx and the other intracellularly. By stimulating the outside of the receptor a message could be passed directly to the interior of the cell.

Pumps composed of enzymes lie within the membrane and on its surfaces.

Receptors, pores and pumps are floating, so to speak, within and on the membrane and are an integral part of it. They can be withdrawn, repaired, replaced, concentrated and altered, thereby changing the response pattern of the cell. This is the 'mosaic model' of the plasma membrane.

THE CELL

Activity

The plasma membrane can bind molecules or larger bodies to its inner or outer surfaces and retain them, or react to them, or transfer them from one side to the other.

It is obviously necessary for a plasma membrane to be able to recognize those molecules the cell requires for its internal metabolism and those the cell needs to reject either because they are waste products or because they have been manufactured and need to be transferred outside for the benefit of other cells. Proteinaceous receptors bind to such molecules, and enzyme systems transfer them through the membrane which then releases them on the other side.

Cells also need to recognize other cells particularly those which can move through the tissues such as macrophages and fibroblasts, and those which need to react in induction/differentiation processes or to aggregate during embryogenesis. Once again, proteins or glycoproteins associated with the plasma membrane and glycocalyx are involved. Reactions are probably initiated by an interaction caused by the two proteins binding together.

Larger bodies or aggregations of molecules are treated differently. During pinocytosis (fluid ingress) and phagocytosis (particle ingress) the plasma membrane sends out processes (?a reaction initiated by protein receptors) which surround and engulf the molecular aggregate (*Fig. 2.1*). The resulting membrane-bound aggregate is passed into the cell where it is metabolized.

This process is reversed when membrane-bound molecular aggregates (contained in vesicles) are passed out of the cell. The membrane of the vesicle unites with the plasma membrane which subsequently ruptures and discharges its contents extracellularly (*Fig. 2.1*). This activity is known as exocytosis.

Origin and Turnover

It is clear that plasma membrane must be formed during mitosis and the growth of cells, and that it must be replaced following pinocytosis during which a part of the membrane is used to surround the ingested material. If its membrane could not grow a cell would become progressively smaller. Mechanisms therefore exist to insert and remove plasma membrane. During reverse pinocytosis the plasma membrane lengthens and later needs to be trimmed. It also appears that even in the absence of such activities, the plasma membrane and the glycocalyx are constantly being renewed.

A hypothesis, supported by observations, is that phospholipids are synthesized in nuclear and rough endoplasmic reticulum (RER) membranes. Some of these phospholipids are detached as collapsed vesicles and are later inserted into plasma membranes. The phospholipids contained in vesicles which have collapsed after discharging their contents into the cytoplasm (following pinocytosis for example) are recirculated back to the plasma membrane.

Attachments

Some cells, such as those constituting all epithelia, stick together while others, such as fibroblasts, tend to separate from each other. All cells have charged surfaces which tend to repel each other with the result that specialized connections are required to maintain contacts between them. These are tight junctions (*zonulae occludentes*), adhesive zones (*zonulae adherentes*), desmosomes (*maculae adherentes*) and gap junctions (*nexuses*).

Tight Junctions

These effectively seal intercellular spaces. The 20 nm wide glycocalyx is lost and the two adjacent layers of plasma membrane fuse with each other (*Fig. 2.3a*) to produce a three-layered structure. To seal epithelial cells together and prevent material passing, for example, directly from the gut lumen into the underlying mesoderm, tight junctions must (and do) form belts surrounding the whole periphery of each cell.

Adhesive Zones

These attachment zones also form continuous belts but the normal 20 nm gap between cells is maintained. An electron-dense fibrillar mat lies against the intracellular side of the plasma membrane.

Desmosomes

These are the most complex of the cellular connections. The gap between adjacent cell membranes is widened to 25 nm and contains electron-dense material. A layer of dense cytoplasm, the attachment plaque, is separated from the inner surface of the plasma membrane by a lucid layer. Tonofibrils radiate into the cell from the attachment plaque. Desmosomes are 'spot' contacts or 'studs' rather than belts (*Fig 2.3c*).

Junctional Complex

This complex joins the apical ends of adjacent cells in many glandular epithelia and, in the context of dental histology, both proximal and distal ends of ameloblasts, for example. Passing from the proximal end of the cell a junctional complex consists of tight junction (belt), adhesive zone (belt) and desmosomes (a ring of spot contacts) (*Fig. 2.3d*).

THE CELL

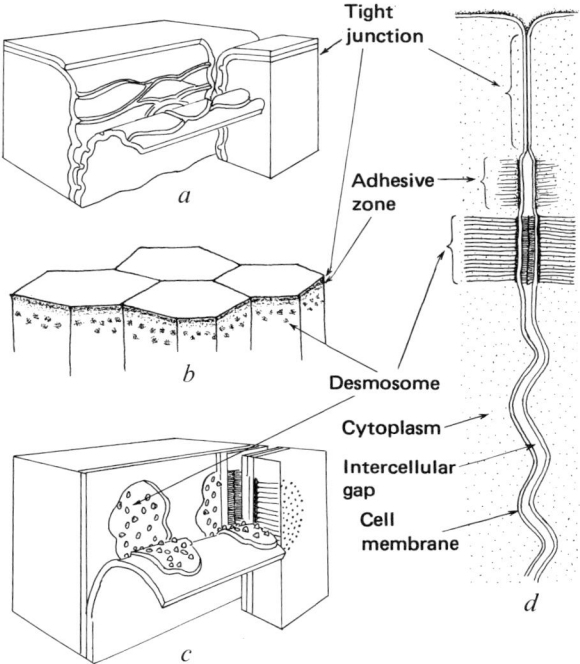

Fig. 2.3. Types of cell attachment. (After Warwick R. and Williams P. L. in *Gray's Anatomy*.) *a* and *c* are three-dimensional representations. *b* shows the ends of four cells. *d* is the appearance of cell contacts in an electron micrograph.

Terminal Bar and Terminal Web

These are terms used in light microscopy. The terminal bar is the bar which apparently joins the ends of adjacent cells in a junctional complex. The electron microscope resolves the bar into the three components of a junctional complex. The terminal web is the spidery array of tonofilaments which radiate out from the desmosomes in the junctional complex.

Gap Junctions

The outer parts of adjacent plasma membranes are separated by about 3 nm in a gap junction. These are spot contacts between cells, rather than continuous belts, and allow ions to pass from cell to cell thereby providing electrical continuity between all the cells in a layer.

Shape

The shape of the cell surface is presumably determined by intra- and extra-cellular pressures and attachments, and by the properties of the membrane itself. For example, the stellate cells in the stellate reticulum are probably compressed due to the pressure exerted by water adsorbed by the surrounding proteoglycans, but remain attached to each other by desmosomes. *Microvilli* each contain a fibrillar core which attaches a villus to the underlying cell web (*Fig. 2.1*). The development of a *pseudopodium* is related to forces developed in the cytoplasm possibly in relation to the assembly of a scaffolding of microfilaments.

NUCLEUS

The nuclear envelope is a double membrane which is continuous with cisternae of endoplasmic reticulum from which it seems to be derived (*Fig. 2.1*). The karyoplasm (the contents of the nucleus) is continuous with the cytoplasm through nuclear pores which account for about 10 per cent of the surface area of the nuclear membrane. The inner layer of the nuclear membrane appears attached to nuclear chromatin; possibly the chromosomes are anchored in this way and prevented from escaping into the cytoplasm. It is probable that the size of the nuclear pores can be varied in order to control the passage of materials to and from the nucleus.

Chromosomal DNA needs little description in this text. Some of the DNA is uncoiled and active (the extended form) while some is coiled and inactive (the condensed form). The DNA is associated with proteins, many of which are enzymes, controlling the activity of the DNA. The DNA is 'naked' inert information expressed in one dimension—a linear sequence of nucleotides. Although convenient it is, strictly speaking, inaccurate to speak of DNA activity. The activity is associated with enzymes which are themselves activated or inactivated by molecules passing in and out of the nucleus through the nuclear pores.

A nucleolus is a roughly spherical, basophilic structure in the karyoplasm and is the region where ribosomal RNA (r-RNA) is synthesized. A nucleus may contain several nucleoli. A loop of DNA passes into the nucleolus from a part of the chromosome known as a nucleolar organizer. Within the nucleolus, the loop of DNA is surrounded by proteins associated with the manufacture of r-RNA. From the nucleolus, the manufactured r-RNA is passed into the cytoplasm through nuclear pores. Messenger RNA (m-RNA) and transfer RNA (t-RNA) are developed from nuclear DNA not associated with the nucleolus. Both require processing before they enter the cytoplasm in active forms.

THE CELL
PROTEIN SYNTHESIS
Ribosomes

Ribosomes are the organic complexes (about 50 different proteins have been identified with the strands of r-RNA) used to assemble amino-acids into proteins. Either they lie free in the cytoplasm, in which case the protein is retained for use in the cell, or, they line the cisternae of endoplasmic reticulum (*Fig. 2.1*), in which case the protein is subsequently secreted.

With the exception of those in mitochondria, all ribosomes have similar shapes. Each consists of a smaller and a larger subunit separated by a cleft which lodges the m-RNA (*Fig. 2.4*). During protein synthesis, several ribosomes are passing down a (long) strand of m-RNA, the whole unit being known as a polyribosome.

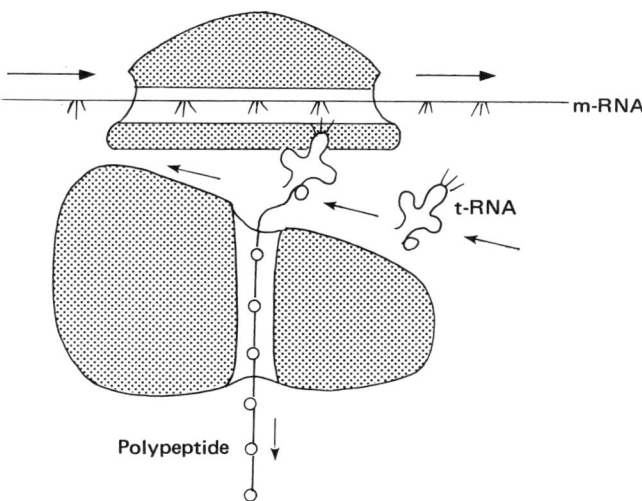

Fig. 2.4. The two parts of a ribosome separated by a cleft.

At the start of protein synthesis the small ribosomal unit attaches to an initiator site on the strand of m-RNA. The large unit is now attached to the small unit to complete the ribosome. An appropriate molecule of transfer RNA, carrying the amino-acid corresponding to the first codon of m-RNA, is captured by the larger subunit of the ribosome. The t-RNA and amino-acid are carried to a second site where the amino-acid is bound and the t-RNA ejected. The m-RNA is moved one step through the ribosome. The next appropriate t-RNA molecule is now captured and transferred to the second site where its amino-acid is linked to the first and the t-RNA ejected. The process is repeated until a 'stop' codon on the m-RNA is reached. The polypeptide has been completed and the ribosome splits into its two units. It takes about 1 minute to link the 150 amino-acid residues of haemoglobin. Since many ribosomes (a polyribosome) are travelling along a strand of m-RNA at the same time the rate of protein synthesis is increased many-fold for each strand of m-RNA.

Endoplasmic Reticulum

Endoplasm is an archaic term referring to the inner cytoplasm. The endoplasmic reticulum is a network (reticulum) which is, in fact, not confined to the endoplasm. It is a system of parallel-sided flattened sacs or cisternae connected to each other and ending at the nuclear membrane (*Fig. 2.1*).

Rough endoplasmic reticulum (RER) is studded with groups of polyribosomes and is associated with the synthesis of proteins for transport out of the cell. The ribosomes are attached to the membrane of the RER, which is similar to the plasma membrane. The folds of the RER membrane may increase its surface area so much that 1 ml of liver tissue has been estimated to contain $7\,m^2$ of RER membrane. Polypeptides synthesized by the polyribosomes are pushed through the membrane and collected in the cisternae where they are assembled into proteins. The proteins, contained in membrane-bound vesicles nipped out of the RER, are then transferred either to the Golgi apparatus or to the plasma membrane (*Fig. 2.1*).

A smooth endoplasmic reticulum, lacking associated ribosomes, is found in some cells (*Fig. 2.1*) which include hepatocytes and intestinal epithelial cells. It is involved in the synthesis of non-protein materials such as lipids and steroids.

Golgi Apparatus

The Golgi apparatus, first demonstrated with light microscopy in 1898, consists of stacks of saucer-shaped saccules (*Fig. 2.1*). The apparatus develops by the aggregation of vesicles, derived from the RER, to form saccules on its convex face. Within the saccules the proteins manufactured by the RER are modified by the addition of carbohydrates, for example. The membranous saccules flow from the (immature) convex side of the Golgi apparatus to the (mature) concave side. Denser vesicles are budded from the mature side and either their contents passed to the extracellular compartment by reverse pinocytosis, or the vesicle is retained in the cell. An important type of vesicle in the latter category is the lysosome.

LYSOSOMES

Lysosomes are organelles which contain hydrolytic enzymes (about 12 have been identified) capable of digesting (lysing) any cellular component. The contents of the cell are protected by isolating these enzymes within membranous sacs. If this membrane is damaged the enzymes are released and attack the cell. Fixation, in formalin for example, stabilizes the lysosomal membranes and prevents autolysis of cells during histological preparation of material.

Primary lysosomes are budded from the mature surface of the Golgi apparatus (*Fig. 2.1*). They contain only hydrolytic enzymes. In order to break down material the primary lysosome fuses with and engulfs material to form a secondary lysosome (phagolysosome). These may be called heterophagosomes if foreign material is ingested, or autophagosomes if part of the cell such as an effete mitochondrion is ingested.

Peroxisomes

These membrane-bound organelles contain enzymes which oxidize certain substrates, the hydrogen released at the first step being transferred to water to produce hydrogen peroxide. The membrane of the peroxisome isolates the potentially dangerous byproduct, H_2O_2, from the cytoplasm.

MITOCHONDRIA

Most of the functions performed by cells require energy. This is mainly derived from the breakdown of high energy phosphate compounds such as adenosine triphosphate (ATP). Mitochondria are the main source of ATP production.

Mitochondria are ellipsoid organelles with diameters up to about 7 μm. They contain outer and inner membranes which are structurally and functionally different. The outer membrane may have been derived from the ancestral host cell; the inner membrane from an ancestral symbiotic bacterium. The inner membrane is folded into cristae which increases its surface area. Depending on their activity, cells may contain up to one or two thousand mitochondria although ova may contain a quarter of a million. New mitochondria probably arise by fragmentation of the 'parent' and subsequent growth of the fragments. They contain their own DNA and ribosomes which could be involved in such autonomous replication. Old mitochondria are broken down in autophagosomes.

Mitochondria contain some 100 enzymes and co-enzymes arranged in an orderly fashion in and on membranes and compartments. These include the Krebs' cycle enzymes.

Mitochondria can move around cells and may be congregated at specific sites such as in the margin of a striated (salivary) duct or at the basal end of an ameloblast. Their movement would be restricted by intracellular scaffolding.

MICROFILAMENTS (MICROFIBRILS)

Microfilaments are about 10 nm wide and are found in fibroblasts, chondrocytes, nerve cells and many types of epithelia and endodermally derived cells. They contain actin or actin-like proteins and may therefore be able to slide along each other producing contractions equivalent to those of muscle fibres.

Cytochalasin B combines with microfilaments and also inhibits phagocytosis, pinocytosis, reverse pinocytosis, cell movement and the cleavage of cells during mitosis. It is therefore suggested that microfilaments are involved in these processes, all of which involve contractions of the plasma membrane. It can be argued that microfilaments attach to the membrane and from here link with a subjacent 'scaffolding' of other microfilaments. This cytoskeletal framework of cross-linked microfilaments is the stable base from which other microfilaments can pull the plasma membrane into an appropriate shape, such as the equatorial furrow in a dividing cell. A similar framework can, tent-like, support or brace a cell's plasma membrane. This is the probable role of the aggregates of microfilaments which comprise the tonofilaments associated with desmosomes.

MICROTUBULES

Microtubules are hollow cylinders, about 20 nm in diameter, composed of a substance (tubulin) which binds with energy-rich molecules of GTP.

Microtubules are a self-assembling scaffold which provides support for the whole cell. The scaffold is dismantled during mitosis and re-erected as the mitotic spindle which grows out from the centrioles and pushes them apart during prophase. Subsequently the microtubules contract during metaphase and pull the chromosomes apart.

The contractile property of microtubules is used to promote cell movement. They are present in the ruffled membrane at the advancing edge of motile cells such as fibroblasts. Cilia and flagellae are composed of them; the tail of a sperm consists of microtubules 70 μm long.

Finally, the microtubular scaffold consists of 'highways' along which substances travel to their appropriate intracellular destinations. The energy for these journeys is derived from the GTP associated with the tubulin. The microtubules in nerve axons and odontoblast processes are associated with the transport of materials.

BASEMENT MEMBRANE AND BASAL LAMINA

For many years light microscopists have recognized that the layer of matrix separating epithelial from mesodermal cells stains heavily with silver. It is called 'basement membrane'. The basement membrane has been analysed in far more detail by biochemical techniques and by electron microscopy.

Basement membrane contains a procollagen-like material (never converted into collagen) which is referred to as type IV collagen. This 'collagen' is combined with non-collagenous material, mainly glycoproteins, the whole biochemical meshwork being probably, but not certainly, derived from the epithelial cells. The fibroblasts adjacent to the basement membrane produce both type I and III collagens and are coated on their surfaces by a further collagen known as type V.

Under the electron microscope three distinct layers appear to separate the epithelial cells from the fibroblasts. Passing from the epithelium, these

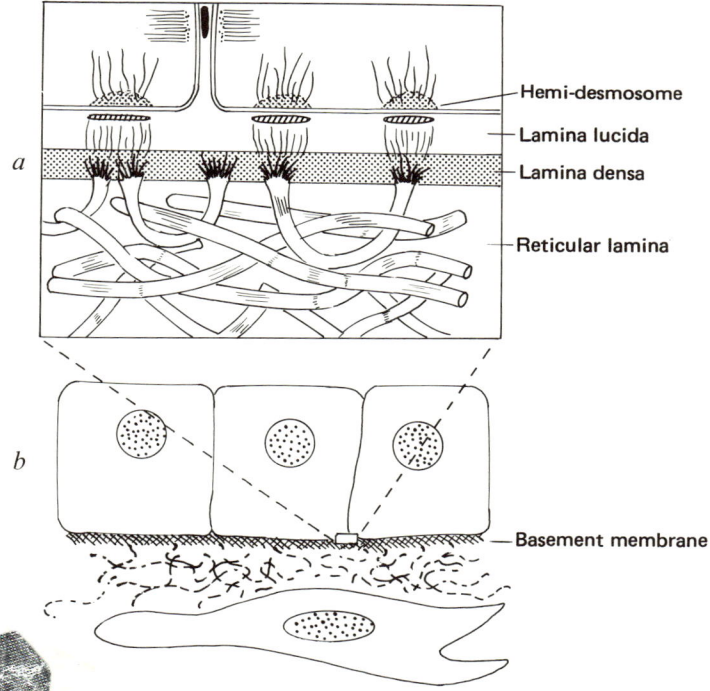

2.5. When a basement membrane seen under the light microscope (*b*) is examined under the electron microscope (*a*) at least three parts can be distinguished. (After Squier A., Johnson N. W. and Hopps R. M. (1976) *Human Oral Mucosa*. Oxford, Blackwell.)

are the lamina lucida and lamina densa, about 0·1 μm wide and collectively termed the basal lamina, and the reticular lamina (*Fig. 2.5*).

Recently it has become possible to equate biochemical findings with the electron microscope appearance of the basal lamina. Thus lamina lucida consists of a glycoprotein the function of which is associated with attachment of epithelial cells. The lamina densa is a sandwich with the bread consisting of heparan sulphate, which determines permeability, and a filling of type IV collagen acting as a structural protein. Type V collagen is associated with the anchoring fibrils.

REFERENCES AND FURTHER READING

Threadgold L. T. (1976) *The Ultrastructure of the Animal Cell*, 2nd ed. Oxford, Pergamon.

Warwick R. and Williams P. L. (1980) *Gray's Anatomy*, 36th ed. Edinburgh, Churchill Livingstone.

The following articles are from the *Scientific American*: A dynamic model of cell membranes. March 1974; The final steps in secretion. October 1975; Junctions between living cells. May 1978; The molecular basis of cell movement. May 1979; The transport of substances in nerve cells. April 1980; Microtubule treadmills. February 1982.

CHAPTER 3

THE TOOTH IN SITU

This brief description of the developing and completed human tooth in situ is meant to introduce the student to the terminology and position of the salient tissues as they might appear in a section of a human jaw. The composite diagrams of *Figs. 3.1* and *3.2* provide a glossary of components rather than an accurate histological picture. The numbers appearing alongside some of the structures and tissues labelled in *Fig. 3.2* refer to the chapter in this book dealing specifically with the features in question, so that the diagrams may also serve as a rapid index.

The forming tooth germ (*Fig. 3.1*) has reached the bell stage of development, during which tissues concerned with crown production are rapidly differentiating.

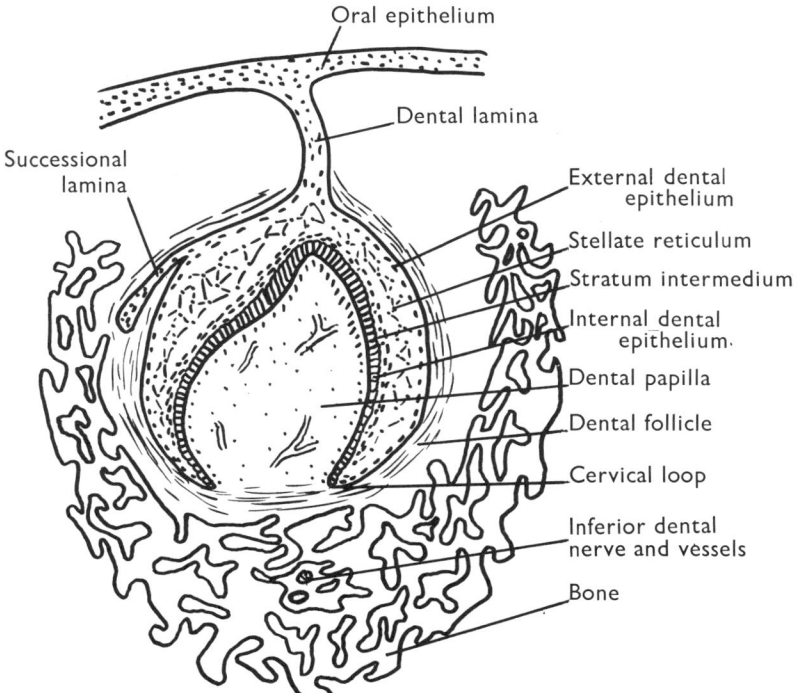

Fig. 3.1. Diagram of a section of a developing tooth in situ.

The dental organ comprises an outer dental epithelium which is continuous with the basal layer of the oral epithelium via the dental lamina. A function of this organ is the production of enamel. At the cervical loop the outer dental epithelium folds sharply and continues over the surface of the papilla as the inner dental epithelium. Adjacent to the inner dental epithelium, and within the dental organ, is a layer of stratified cells forming the stratum intermedium. The dental organ is occupied by a diffuse stellate reticulum which is largely composed of intercellular fluid-filled spaces.

The richly vascular dental papilla contains the many types of cells found in any connective tissue. Its surface is lined by odontoblasts whose chief function is to produce dentine.

Each tooth germ is encapsulated by the dental follicle from which the tooth's supporting tissues are derived.

On the lingual side of the tooth germ, in the region of its attachment to the dental lamina, a successional lamina develops at whose deep edge grows the germ of the permanent tooth.

The nerve and vascular supplies to the tooth germ are derived from main trunks lying beneath its base.

The completed and functional tooth (*Fig. 3.2*) consists of an enamel-covered anatomical crown and a cement-covered anatomical root. The term 'anatomical crown' must be distinguished from the term 'clinical crown'. The clinical crown is that part of the tooth which is exposed in the mouth at any given age. In young persons part of the base of the anatomical crown remains hidden by the gingival margin so that the clinical crown is smaller than the anatomical crown. In elderly persons the gingival margin retreats rootwards (passive eruption), exposing the entire anatomical crown and also often a small portion of the anatomical root. The clinical crown is now larger than the anatomical crown.

The anatomical root is all that part of the tooth lying deep to the level of the cervical margin of the enamel and typically contained within the bony alveolus (socket). Enamel is not normally present on the root except as enamel droplets, commonly found in the root bifurcations of molars.

By far the greatest proportion of a tooth consists of dentine, a mineralized tissue permeated throughout its thickness by regularly arranged dentine tubules, each containing a fine protoplasmic process of an odontoblast cell which is itself situated on the surface of the pulp. The outer surface of the coronal dentine lines the enamel–dentine junction which is microscopically irregular. A further mineralized tissue, cement, lies on the outer surface of the root and serves as an attachment for fibres of the periodontal ligament (*see below*). Immediately beneath the surface of the root dentine there is a microscopically granular layer, termed the 'granular layer of Tomes'. In the centre of the coronal dentine is the pulp chamber which in a young tooth extends as a pulp horn beneath the cusp. A pulp canal runs the entire length of each root and opens into the

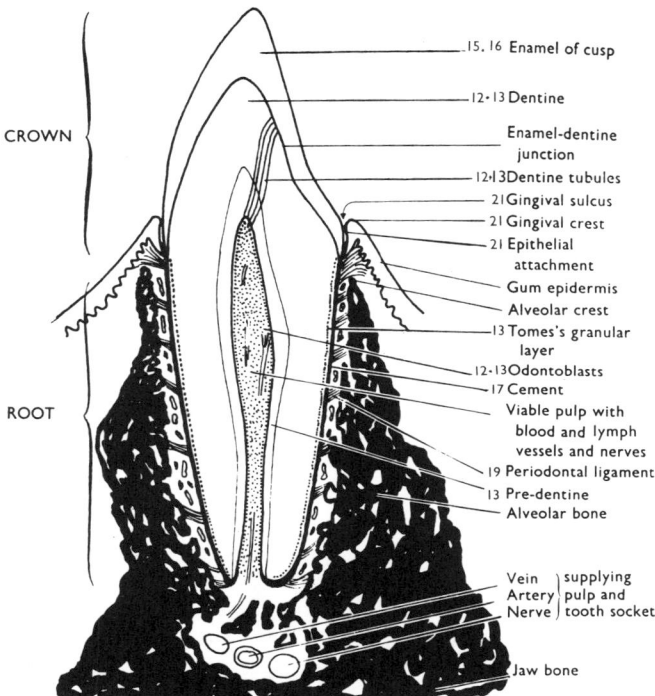

Fig. 3.2. Composite diagram of a longitudinal section of a functional tooth in situ.

periodontal ligament at the apical foramen. The tissue within the pulp cavity is a normal connective tissue covered by specialized cells, the odontoblasts.

Enamel is the refractile microcrystalline, highly mineralized layer on the outer surface of the anatomical crown.

The only site where oral epithelium comes into direct contact with the functional tooth is at the base of the clinical crown. Here the epithelium is turned inwards and attached to the surface of the enamel, producing the gingival sulcus and the epithelial attachment.

The tooth is anchored to its socket in the alveolar bone by the collagen fibres of the periodontal ligament. Most of these fibres run obliquely and coronally from the cement into the alveolar bone. The bundles of fibres which are inserted into the mineralized tissues are called 'Sharpey's fibres'. The term 'alveolar bone' refers to that part of the jaw which contains holes (alveoli). It is not in any way histologically distinguishable from the remaining bone tissue of the jaws. It exists solely to support the teeth and is largely resorbed when the teeth are lost.

CHAPTER 4

THE ROLE OF ECTOMESENCHYME IN TOOTH FORMATION AND INDUCTION

THE NEURAL CREST

Origin

The neural crest, which is the source of ectomesenchyme, is an important primordium found in the early embryo. The fertilized egg rapidly develops to form an embryonic disc consisting of two cell types, an outer layer of ectoderm and an inner layer of endoderm. The space between these two germ layers comes to be occupied by a third germ layer, the mesoderm, thus establishing the trilaminar embryo. At this time the longitudinal axis of the embryo is emphasized by the formation of the neural plate, a symmetrical demarcated area of ectoderm, wider at the future head end, bounded by thickened marginal folds, and extending along the future dorsal surface. In time the neural folds rise up and, approaching each other, meet and fuse along the midline, thus converting the neural plate into a tube which sinks inwards beneath the surface ectoderm (*Fig. 4.1*). During the development of the neural tube small groups of ectodermal cells break away from the margins of the neural plate and come to lie parallel to, and on either side of, the neural tube. These constitute the neural crest cells. It is useful to distinguish between cranial and spinal neural crest.

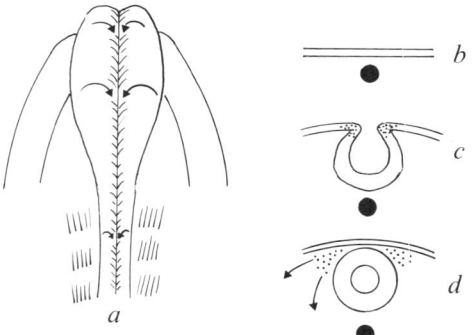

Fig. 4.1. In *a* the developing head end of the neural tube is seen from above. In transverse sections at successive stages of development it can be seen that the notochord (black circle) induces the overlying ectoderm to curl up as the neural tube. Cells from the neural crest (stippled) are pinched out and migrate laterally and dorsally (*Fig. 4.2*).

Significance

Early experiments on salamanders which were continued into the 1940s showed that if the neural folds are removed from particular regions of the neural plate associated with the middle of the developing brain, either teeth or jaw cartilages fail to develop. Later, it was shown for an amphibian that if those neural crest cells, apparently required for tooth development, are transplanted to the abdomen they are able to initiate tooth development. Such experiments indicated that during normal embryogenesis, amphibian neural crest cells either migrate and are themselves transformed to cartilage and tooth-forming cells or they alone have the ability to induce other cells to develop along these lines.

The neural crest cells of amphibians contain a black pigment while their mesodermal cells contain yolk granules. Using this marker, De Beer (1947) demonstrated that odontoblasts in the teeth of embryo salamanders originate from the neural crest. (From other evidence he also showed that in this animal some of the enamel organs originate from ectoderm and others from endoderm.)

Turning now to experiments on birds, the cells of the quail carry natural black markers on their nuclei which can be used to distinguish them from chick cells. A chimera (combination of different animals) consisting of neural plate dissected from a quail embryo combined with a chick embryo from which neural crest has been removed grows in a fairly normal way for some time. Another technique substitutes neural crest tissue (from one chick embryo) which has been soaked in and has taken up a radioactive label for that in another chick embryo. The labelled cells can now be traced in the growing recombined embryo. Both types of experiment indicate that much of the facial skeleton of birds is derived from neural crest (birds, of course, have no teeth).

Experiments on mammals are the most demanding. It has been suggested that neural crest cells can be identified for some time during early development because they contain considerably more RNA than the mesodermal cells with which they are mixing. In serial sections Milaire traced what he supposed to be neural crest cells streaming into the maxillary and mandibular arches of embryo mice (*Fig. 4.2*). The mandibular stream separates into a core apparently associated with the development of Meckel's cartilage and a more peripheral group later associated with tooth development.

The above data destroyed a dogma of embryology which was based on the belief in an early and irrevocable partitioning of the three germ layers: ectoderm, mesoderm and endoderm. The mesoderm, the middle layer of the trilaminar embryo, gives rise to embryonic connective tissue (mesenchyme = the middle juice) from which differentiates a wide range of cells and tissues such as fibrous tissue, tendons, muscle, haemopoietic tissue and so on. The neural crest cells constitute a fourth germ layer which

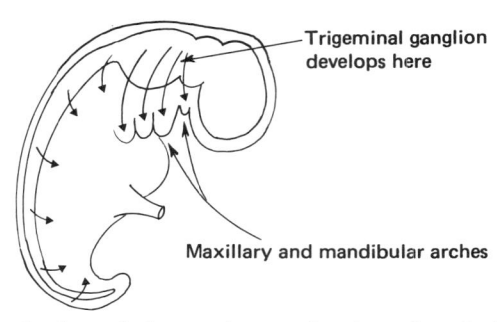

Fig. 4.2. From head to tail the neural crest cells migrate into the branchial arches and through the body.

migrates away from the neural tube and mingles with the derivatives of both ectoderm and mesoderm. In association with ectoderm the neural crest cells differentiate to become the pigment cells of the skin, the cranial, spinal and autonomic ganglia of the nervous system (including obviously those of V, VII and IX) and their associated Schwann cells, and the adrenal medulla. In the cranial region the neural crest cells contribute the meninges and much of the cartilage and bone of the facial skeleton, tissues which at one time were thought to arise from the mesoderm. In order to distinguish between the origins of mesodermal cells they can be referred to as endomesenchyme (mesodermal origin) and ectomesenchyme (neural crest origin).

From the above data it became clear that apart from their contribution to the development of the nervous system, the neural crest cells in their ectomesenchyme role are transformed into the chondroblasts and osteoblasts from which develop the cartilages and bones of the facial region and into the odontoblasts from which dentine develops.

INDUCTION, COMPETENCE AND DIFFERENTIATION

At any stage in development it is possible to trace the ancestry of a cell back to the zygote. Each cell belongs to a lineage in which successive generations differ to a greater or lesser degree, or not at all, from adjacent generations. Differences can be categorized as those in (1) metabolic profile, (2) shape and (3) rate of cell division. Any set of these parameters describes a particular *compartment* in which a cell exists. Movement into a new compartment is known as *differentiation*.

A cell lineage may continue in the same compartment until acted on by a stimulus, following which the daughter cells enter a new compartment: for example, they may start producing a new protein, change their shape or stop dividing. The process which induces the change is known as *induction* and the cells are *induced* to differentiate.

It has often been observed that the response of a population of embryonic cells changes with time. The *competence* of the population to react to an inducing agent gradually increases to a maximum and then falls to zero. What changes the competence of a cell line? Since the members of the line are first unable to react, are then capable of reacting and finally fail to react, they must be changing compartments. Such differentiation may often be autonomous and not involve an external inducing agent. For other lines the change may require induction from a different cell line.

The requirements for differentiation are probably varied. The cell must be competent to react. Competence may involve the possession of cell surface receptors (*see Fig. 2.2*) which can respond either to a substance in the environment which is secreted by an inducer cell or to physical contact with the cell membrane of the inducer cell. The 'activated' receptor now initiates a cytoplasmic response which is transferred to the nucleus where a new activity is initiated. The cell differentiates.

Cells may be competent to react, but never receive the necessary inducer stimulus. Kollar and Fisher (1980) cultured oral epithelium from embryo chicks with dental ectomesenchyme from the jaws of embryo mice. Teeth developed from the combination. The chick epithelial cells expressed the competence to partake in tooth development, an activity last expressed by birds over 100 million years ago in the fossil *Hesperornis*. Chick oral epithelium cells seem to have maintained the competence to form an enamel organ but they are never induced during normal embryogenesis. (However, it is just possible that a few mouse epithelial cells may have contaminated the culture and these later multiplied and differentiated into the enamel organ.)

In the same way, certain cells may maintain the ability to induce differentiation but the respondents have lost the competence to react.

EPITHELIAL/MESENCHYMAL INTERACTIONS

A whole class of inductive events between epithelium and the underlying connective tissue cells are referred to as epithelial/mesenchymal interactions. These have been studied by separating the tissues and recombining and culturing them *in vitro* separated by a very thin, inert and porous membrane. By changing the size of the pores in the membrane and by studying any cell processes or materials which enter the pores it is possible to investigate the nature of the inductive stimulus.

Presumptive salivary mesenchyme (mesenchyme which will later be incorporated as the supporting tissue of the salivary gland) on one side of the porous membrane induces presumptive salivary epithelium on the other side of the membrane to differentiate into glandular salivary epithelium. Without this mesenchyme the presumptive salivary epithelium does not differentiate and soon degenerates. Ordinary jaw mesenchyme cannot induce the differentiation, but its presence prevents the epithelium from degenerating. Finally, if presumptive pancreatic epithelium is associated with the salivary gland mesenchyme, pancreatic glandular cells are differentiated.

The above experiments suggest the existence of three types of epithelial/mesenchymal interactions.

1. Epithelial tissues require an underlying mesenchyme if they are to be maintained and not degenerate. In the absence of any further knowledge this is known as 'mesodermal maintenance factor'.

2. Some mesenchyme appears able to dictate to an overlying epithelium the path along which to differentiate. As a further example in this category, dental papilla cells can induce the development of a dental organ from (*a*) oral epithelium which would normally co-operate in tooth development, (*b*) from oral epithelium which would not normally take part in tooth development (e.g. diastema epithelium from rodent jaws and the chick oral epithelium referred to above), (*c*) from abdominal epithelium (the experiment referred to above) and (*d*) from foot epithelium. In all these cases the epithelium must, obviously, be competent to respond. It can be argued that such competence is not due to the acquisition of specific receptors, because so many different epithelia are able to respond, but resides in some potency of the inducing cells. Alternatively it is interesting that teeth almost certainly evolved from the dermal denticles of ancestral fish. It might therefore be argued that embryonic skin (and oral) epithelia still pass through a stage during which they develop the specific ancestral receptors to react to tooth induction by dental mesenchyme.

3. Some apparently undifferentiated epithelia already occupy a (differentiation) compartment along a specified lineage. Mesenchyme from foreign sources can trigger an epithelial receptor which initiates a predetermined response; no matter what the nature of the induction, the response is always the same. In this case it can be visualized that the actual molecules responsible for intitiating the change in nuclear activity are attached inside the cell's plasma membrane. An inductive event outside the cell causes these molecules to be released and passed to the nucleus. A large number of very different stimuli might produce the same inductive event. The only characteristic they need have in common is an ability to cause the 'inductive' molecule to be released from inside the plasma membrane.

ROLE OF ECTOMESENCHYME INTERACTIONS INVOLVING NEURAL CREST CELLS

It is only after they have migrated into the branchial arches that neural crest cells become *scleroblasts*, a collective term used to describe cells forming mineralized tissues or cartilage. At what stage in their development can cranial neural crest cells become scleroblasts, and what induces their differentiation?

It appears that before they can progress towards differentiation as scleroblasts, neural crest cells must first be induced by a proliferating epithelium. In birds this potentiating interaction takes place before the neural crest cells migrate away from the developing neural tube and may be related to the overlying ectoderm; in amphibians it is later and involves pharyngeal endoderm; in mammals it is later still and involves oral epithelium.

It will be recalled that mammalian neural crest divides into two streams inside the mandibular arch. The central core of neural crest cells interacts at a distance with proliferating oral epithelium and from it differentiate the chondroblasts of Meckel's cartilage. Later, osteoblasts differentiate from a clump of these neural crest cells lateral to Meckel's cartilage and begin the development of the bony mandible. The peripheral stream of neural crest lies directly under the oral epithelium. These cells induce the overlying epithelium to proliferate more rapidly and grow into the jaws as the dental lamina (*see* Chapter 5). It may be that contact with pioneer nerve fibres is also necessary to induce the appearance of the dental lamina. The neural crest cells now interact with dental lamina to produce discrete tooth germs which become surrounded by dental follicles derived from the remaining cells of the peripheral stream of neural crest.

REFERENCES AND FURTHER READING

De Beer G. R. (1947) The differentiation of neural crest cells into odontoblasts in ambystoma and re-examination of the germ-layer theory. *Proc. R. Soc.* **134-B**, 377.

Cummings E. G., Bringas P. B., Grodin M. S. et al. (1981) Epithelial-directed mesenchyme differentiation *in vitro*. *Differentiation* **20**, 1.

Fleischmajer R. and Billingham R. E. (1968) *Epithelial–Mesenchymal Interactions.* Baltimore, Williams & Wilkins.

Gaunt W. A. (1959) The vascular supply to the dental lamina during early development. *Acta Anat.* **37**, 232.

Gaunt W. A. and Miles A. E. W. (1967) Fundamental aspects of tooth morphogenesis. In: Miles A. E. W. (ed.), *Structural and Chemical Organization of Teeth*, vol. 1. New York, Academic.

Hall B. K. (1978) *Developmental and Cellular Skeletal Biology.* New York, Academic.

Kollar E. J. and Baird G. R. (1970a) Tissue interactions in embryonic mouse tooth germs. *J. Emb. Exp. Morphol* **24**, 159.

Kollar E. J. and Baird G. R. (1970b) Tissue interactions in embryonic mouse tooth germs. *J. Emb. Exp. Morphol* **24**, 173.
Kollar E. J. and Fisher C. (1980) Tooth induction in chick epithelium: expression of quiescent genes for enamel synthesis. *Science* **207**, 993.
Slavkin H. C. and Bavetta L. A. (1972) *Developmental Aspects of Oral Biology*. New York, Academic.

CHAPTER 5

THE EARLY DEVELOPMENT OF THE TEETH

It is not intended to give here a detailed account of the histological changes which have been observed during development of the human tooth. The reader is referred to standard texts for complete details.

The epithelium in the front of the mouth is derived from the lining of the original invaginated stomatodeum and is accordingly of ectodermal origin. Further back in the mouth the oral lining is derived from the endoderm of the embryonic pharynx, though the precise line of demarcation is controversial (*Fig. 5.1*). Certainly, there is no detectable histological distinction between the front and the back of the mouth where the buccopharyngeal membrane has broken down.

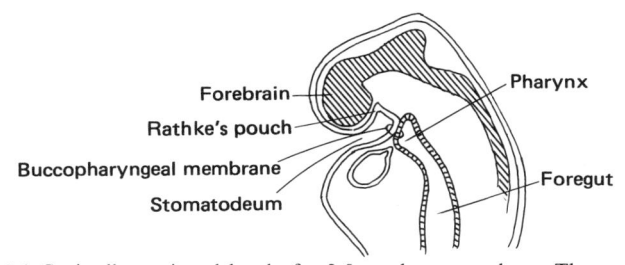

Fig. 5.1. Sagittally sectioned head of a 2·5 mm human embryo. The central nervous system and the (endodermal) lining of the alimentary canal are shaded.

Knowledge of the very early development of the dentition is confused and uncertain. At about 8 weeks in human development a stage is reached where, around the whole of what will subsequently be the dental arch, the oral epithelium bulges into the underlying mesoderm. This horseshoe-shaped thickening is the *dental lamina*. Adjacent to it the underlying mesodermal cells, which have travelled from the neural crest, are more concentrated than elsewhere (*Fig. 5.2*). The confusion relates to the sequence of changes which lead to this stage of development.

DENTAL LAMINA

The first signs of dental development are the appearance of localized thickenings of oral ectoderm in each subsequent incisor and molar

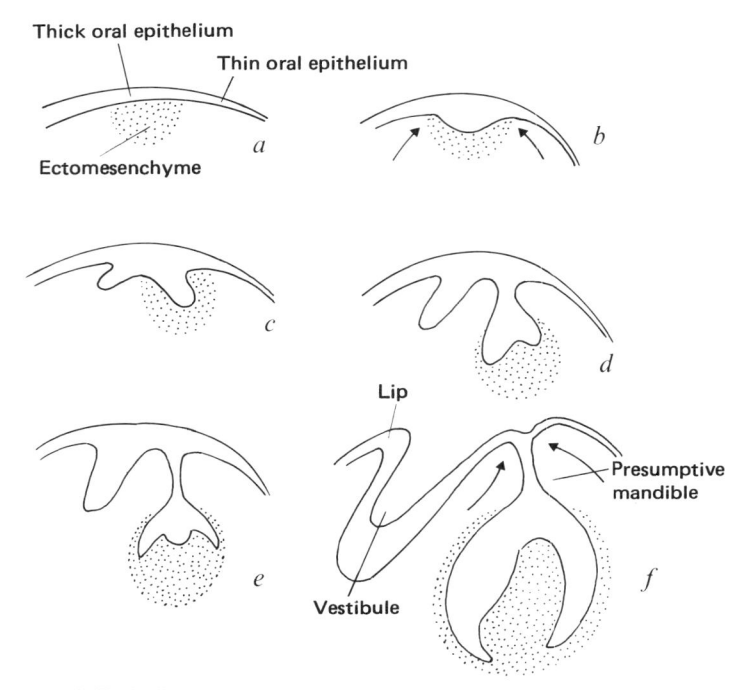

Fig. 5.2. Each diagram represents a sagittal section of the skull through the subsequent incisor region.

a, Ectomesenchyme is concentrated beneath the thick pharyngeal epithelium which covers the subsequent tooth bearing region of the jaw. The lip will be to the left. *b*, The formation of the primary epithelial band. *c*, The vestibular band pushes anteriorly into the adjacent mesenchyme while the dental lamina grows into the ectomesenchyme. *d*, A tooth bud forms at the end of the dental lamina. The vestibular band increases in size. *e*, The ectodermal part of the tooth bud extends around the growing ball of ectomesenchymal cells to produce a cap. *f*, Continued growth of the ectodermal cells around the growing ball of ectomesenchymal cells results in a bell-shaped enamel organ. The central cells of the vestibular band break down separating a lip on the left from the subsequent alveolar region of the jaw on the right.

region—two in each jaw quadrant. Kollar and Lumsden (1979) relate the epithelial thickening in the molar region of the mouse to the advent of the terminal twig of a nerve axon which (almost?) touches the overlying epithelium. Following this induction the epithelium thickens locally and the underlying mesoderm condenses. An alternative is that the ectomesenchymal cells induce the appearance of the dental lamina. In support of this view, no nerve has been shown in the incisor region of induction.

The incisal and molar regions of thickened epithelium spread anteriorly and posteriorly. This spread could be due either to the conversion of intervening epithelial cells into dental lamina or to the expanding growth of the two clumps of cells. In rodents the intervening cells do not differentiate into dental lamina. No teeth develop here, this naturally occurring edentulous region being known as a diastema. In man Ooë (1981) has demonstrated the spread of dental lamina from two regions in each upper and lower jaw quadrant with a transient hiatus between the incisor and canine regions. Finally, the dental lamina unites around the whole jaw.

The dental lamina now deepens into the underlying mesoderm. It does not appear to grow downwards because Osman and Ruch (1975) have shown that there is no increase in the mitotic activity of the lamina as opposed to the epithelial cells on its buccal and lingual sides. The only alternative seems to be that the mesoderm on each side of the lamina grows orally pushing upwards and pinching together the epithelium on each side of the lamina thereby deepening it (*Fig. 5.2*).

VESTIBULAR LAMINA

In the next stage of development a band of epithelium lateral to the dental lamina grows into the mesoderm. This is the *vestibular lamina*. It is not clear whether the vestibular lamina is independent of the dental lamina or whether it is an outgrowth from the dental lamina. If the latter is the correct interpretation of the appearances, the initial epithelial invagination should be referred to as the *primary epithelial band* and the terms 'dental lamina' and 'vestibular lamina' restricted to its two extensions.

TOOTH BUDS

Ectomesenchymal cells now begin clumping beneath the dental lamina in regions which correspond with the later appearance of teeth. These initiate the development of tooth buds. Several theories have been proposed to account for their distribution.

The sites at which tooth buds are initiated might be determined by an earlier equivalent pattern in the distribution of either capillaries or nerves. The first explanation is based on the pattern of capillaries present in the jaws of the cat prior to the appearance of tooth buds (Gaunt and Miles, 1967). The second is based on two lines of evidence. It has been shown in histological studies that the site at which each vibrissa on a mouse develops can be predicted from the distribution of developing nerve terminals. Nerves seem to have the same determining effect on the location of taste buds. By extrapolation, the same may be true for tooth buds: twigs of the branching trigeminal nerve each cause the initiation of a tooth germ. The other line of evidence is described above and relates to the nerve twig associated with the initiation of the molar dental lamina in mice.

Against the above interpretations lies the observation that if a very early first molar bud from an embryo mouse is removed and cultured in the anterior chamber of the eye, all three molar teeth develop (Lumsden 1979). It is almost impossible to conceive that the anterior chamber of the eye contains the same pattern of capillaries or nerve twigs that develop in the mandible of an embryo. Incidentally, if nerves initiate each tooth bud the problem of the distribution of tooth buds is merely transferred into the problem of the distribution of nerve terminals.

It has next been proposed that some sort of signal, chemical or electrical, arises at the front of the jaw, passes back and initiates the development of teeth. Such theories come under the general heading of 'field theories'.

A final theory is loosely based on the concept of cell clones (Osborn, 1978). A group of identical cells is known as a clone. The dentition in each jaw quadrant is supposed to develop from three clones of ectomesenchymal cells: *incisor, canine* and *molar clones*. The molar clone in man, for example, is sited in the region of the first deciduous molar and, together with the adjacent dental lamina which it has induced to co-operate in tooth development, grows posteriorly by means of a *progress zone* at its posterior margin (*Fig. 5.3*). When the clone has reached a critical size a tooth bud is initiated at its centre. From this time onwards the clone is constantly poised to initiate new buds but is prevented by a zone of inhibition which temporarily surrounds every newly initiated bud. When the progress zone has grown posteriorly beyond the zone of inhibition a new bud is initiated, and so on until the progress zone ceases growing. This theory achieved support when it was shown that the bud of a mouse

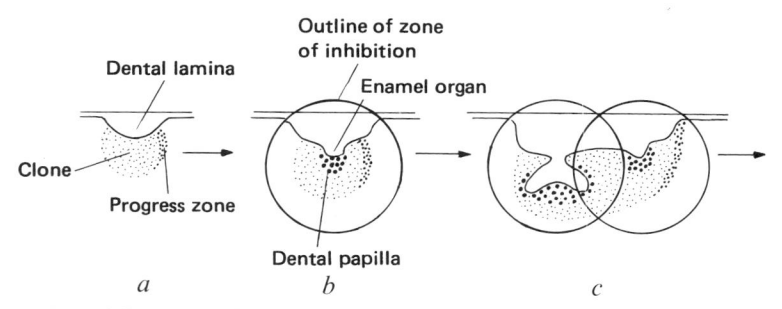

Fig. 5.3. By means of its progress zone (medium stipple) the clone cells (light stipple) in *a* grow to become those in *c*, at the same time inducing the co-operation of the overlying oral ectoderm. The central cells differentiate to become dental papillae. As soon as a tooth bud appears, it becomes surrounded by a zone in which the differentiation of a new papilla is temporarily inhibited.

first molar (together with some adherent cells) developed all three molar teeth when grown in the anterior chamber of the eye away from any signals or tissues present in the developing mandible. Presumably the first molar bud lies in the centre of the early molar clone of the mouse and the clone grows posteriorly.

CONDENSATIONS OF CELLS

It is not known what causes the ectomesenchymal cells to condense beneath the dental lamina and the early tooth buds. First, this could be due to more rapid cell division, but measurements suggest the cells are not dividing more rapidly. Second, cells could migrate towards foci and produce condensations. Third, the core of the branchial arch is expanding outwards due to the production of extracellular material with the result that in most regions, despite a limited rate of mitosis, the cells are not becoming more concentrated. If little extracellular material is being produced at the foci representing early tooth buds the dividing cells will not separate and therefore appear to be condensed in relation to the rest of the mesoderm.

TOOTH FOLLICLE

Two or three weeks after a discrete (deciduous) tooth bud has been initiated, the bone of the developing jaw spreads towards the oral cavity and begins to isolate each tooth germ within a bony crypt which, in the dried skull, is open to the oral cavity. The soft tissue between the tooth and the wall of the crypt was for long known as the tooth follicle (*see Fig. 3.2*) but this terminology has recently been changed (Chapter 19). Within the follicle the developing tooth is able to undergo slight positional adjustments caused by growth forces generated by its developing crown. The inner layer of this soft tissue reinforces the tooth germ preventing it being distorted and also gives origin to the periodontal ligament.

Replacement teeth (the permanent incisors and canines and the premolars) are almost completely surrounded by their bony crypts (*see Fig. 3.1*). The tooth follicle is continuous with the lamina propria of the oral mucosa above through a hole in the crypt, the *gubernacular canal*. This canal contains fibrous tissue and remnants of the dental lamina together known as the *gubernacular cord*. The (ectodermal) tissue of the dental lamina may be responsible for preventing bone sealing the bony crypt around the (permanent) successional teeth.

GROWTH OF THE TOOTH GERM

A *tooth germ* is the structure from which a tooth is developed. Three early stages are recognized: the bud, cap and bell stages (*Fig. 5.2*).

Tooth Bud

Each tooth bud consists of a ball of ectomesenchymal cells, the *dental papilla*, topped by an expansion of ectodermal (or endodermal) cells, the *dental organ*, which is continuous with the dental lamina.

The dental organ and dental papilla proliferate and grow. A mechanism must exist to control the directions in which the dental organ grows because throughout development, including that of the root, its surface and derivatives (the root sheath) remain in contact with the growing surface of the dental papilla. Some form of *contact guidance* may be involved whereby cells in the opposing surface layers have receptors which maintain them in contact with the basement membrane which separates them.

Cap Stage

The dental organ grows faster than the dental papilla with the result that it spreads over the surface of the papilla and takes on the appearance of a cap. This is the cap stage of development (*Fig. 5.2e*). Some of the dental papilla cells are pushed aside and come to lie on the outer surface of the enamel organ. These cells comprise an *investing layer* or more properly the tooth follicle.

During the cap stage histodifferentiation begins. As the dental organ grows, its innermost cells become increasingly separated from the vascular tissues in the dental papilla and tooth follicle. The central cells begin secreting glycosaminoglycans (GAGS) into the narrow intercellular spaces which separate them (*Fig. 5.4a*). These GAGS are intensely hydrophilic and water is pulled into the intercellular spaces, compressing the cytoplasm of each of the cells within the inner mass (*Fig. 5.4b*). All the cells of the dental organ are united by desmosomes and despite the compression of their cytoplasm the desmosomal connections between the inner cells are maintained. This process results in the development of a stellate reticulum whose intercellular spaces are filled with water and GAGS.

Owing to the appearance of intercellular fluid-filled spaces, the stellate reticulum swells into a turgid diffuse tissue whose functions may be considered under two headings, mechanical and nutritional. In a mechanical sense, it has been suggested that the stellate reticulum serves to protect the developing tooth germ against mechanical disturbance from without, and to provide the requisite space for the crown to develop within the

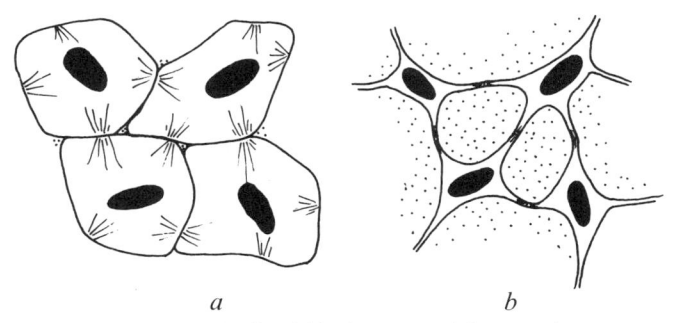

Fig. 5.4. a, Four polygonal cells within the centre of the enamel organ secrete glycosaminoglycans (stippled) into the intercellular region. The glycosaminoglycans are hydrophilic and water is absorbed (*b*). The desmosomal connections between the cells are maintained producing the stellate reticulum.

tooth follicle. It has also been suggested that the tissue's turgor pressure serves to maintain the spherical shape of the dental organ during development and at the same time to balance the growth pressures generated by the expanding dental papilla (ectomesenchyme). In terms of nutrition the GAGS within the stellate reticulum steadily diminish during enamel formation. Perhaps their role, and that of the stellate reticulum, is to contribute to the development of the enamel matrix.

The epithelial cells adjacent to the ectomesenchyme become cuboidal and then low columnar in shape, the layer being now called the 'inner dental epithelium'. The cells of the outer dental epithelium remain roughly cuboidal. They meet the inner dental epithelium at the *cervical loop*, the growing rim of the dental organ, which is streaming over the surface of the dental papilla.

During the cap stage the centre of the inner dental epithelium expands, due to mitosis, into a mass of cells which bulges into the dental papilla and is known as the *enamel knot* (*Fig. 5.2e*). Its role is unknown but it appears to contribute cells to another structure known as the enamel cord (*see later*).

Bell Stage

The mass of ectomesenchymal cells continues to increase in size but the steady encircling action of the dental organ also continues until it surrounds such a large part of the dental papilla that the tooth germ takes on the appearance of a bell—the bell stage of tooth development (*see Figs. 3.1 and 5.2f*). During this stage the major cusps, ridges and fissures of the ultimate crown pattern are established by the development of folds in the inner dental epithelium. The dynamics of the folding process form the subject of the next chapter.

At the early bell stage of development a new layer of cells known as the *stratum intermedium* differentiates within the enamel organ between the inner dental epithelium and the stellate reticulum. It is about three or four cells thick, the cells being compressed and flattened against the inner dental epithelium. Presumably this layer is derived from the cells inside the dental organ, perhaps from the diminishing enamel knot. The suggestion has been made that cells of the stratum intermedium may insinuate between the cells of the inner dental epithelium helping to increase the surface area of this encircling layer. It seems more probable that their only function is to manufacture materials which are passed to the ameloblasts and thence, presumably, into the enamel matrix.

During the bell stage the stellate reticulum often becomes partially or totally divided by a cord of cells extending from the enamel knot, where it is associated with the stratum intermedium, and up to the outer dental epithelium. This structure is the *enamel cord* or, if it completely divides the stellate reticulum, the *enamel septum*. The outer dental epithelium is invaginated into an *enamel navel* where it meets the enamel septum (*see Fig. 15.1a*). The enamel cord overlies the position at which the incisal edge of the first cusp of a tooth is developed. Its function is obscure. It may act as a source of cells for the stellate reticulum or as a mechanical tie across the centre of the dental organ—but it is not always present.

DENTAL AND VESTIBULAR LAMINAE (CONCLUSION)

At about 11 weeks of development, when bony crypts are beginning to grow up around the deciduous tooth germs, a new extension grows lingually from the dental lamina. This is the *successional lamina* (*see Fig. 3.1*) from which develop the tooth germs of the permanent incisors and canines and the premolars. The successional lamina is continuous around the jaw arch and where it is adjacent to tooth germs arises from somewhere near the junction between the dental lamina and the outer dental epithelium.

As a deciduous tooth germ enlarges it appears to move deeper into the jaw with the result that the dental lamina lengthens. Either the tooth germ is growing into the jaws or, what seems more likely, the ectomesenchymal tissues are growing and pushing the oral epithelium into the oral cavity away from the tooth germ thereby deepening the lamina (*Fig. 5.2*). The latter explanation is consistent with the observation that the lamina breaks into fragments, as if it were being disrupted by stretching, and degenerates. The degenerating epithelium forms concentric nests of cells which may keratinize in their centres before finally dying. These are known as 'cell pearls', 'cell nests' or 'cell whorls'. They may later become cystic.

Behind the second deciduous molar the dental lamina burrows backwards without a connection with the oral epithelium. The permanent molars are successively budded from its growing end.

The vestibular lamina grows into the ectomesenchyme lateral to the developing dentition. Alternatively, as with the dental lamina, the ectomesenchyme pushes orally on each side of the vestibular lamina. The central epithelial cells die and a vestibule is formed buccal to the developing teeth and alveolar bone (*Fig. 5.2*).

SEQUENCES OF TOOTH DEVELOPMENT

Human permanent upper teeth develop in the sequence 1, 6, 2, 4, 3, 5, 7, 8. The mole, for example, has 11 maxillary teeth and they are initiated in the sequence 1, 4, 8, 7, 2, 6, 3, 9, 10, 5, 11. How might such sequences, which are clearly genetically determined, be controlled? Only one solution has been suggested.

The mole dentition contains 3 incisors, 1 canine, 4 premolars and 3 molars. The clone model proposes (Osborn, 1978) that each quadrant of a mammalian dentition consists of three different clones of mesodermal (ectomesenchymal) cells: incisor, canine and molar clones. Consider an incisor clone (*Fig. 5.5*). The primordial clone of identical cells interacts with oral epithelium and generates a growing mass of potential tooth-forming tissue. In this case the clone grows by means of a *progress zone* situated posteriorly (*Fig. 5.3*). As soon as a critical mass is achieved a tooth primordium is initiated at its centre. The primordium generates around it a zone in which the initiation of a further primordium is temporarily inhibited. A new tooth is initiated when the posterior progress zone has grown beyond this inhibitory zone. This cycle continues until the clone ceases growing. The same explanation can be used to describe the

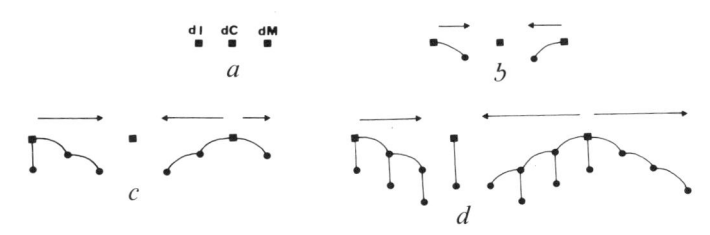

Fig. 5.5. The jaws of eutherian mammals are supposed to contain three developmental segments; incisor, canine and molar (*d*). The teeth in each segment are budded in sequence from three 'stem' tooth families (*a*). These sequences (*a–d*) determine the gradients in tooth shape. Squares represent the 'stem' tooth buds; circles represent teeth; vertical lines connect deciduous teeth with their replacements; the arcs connect deciduous teeth of the same segment.

initiation of the permanent incisors by means of an inferior progress zone. Those clone cells not incorporated in tooth primordia (and the investing layer of the follicle) contribute the periodontium surrounding each tooth. The number of teeth which develop is related to the size the clone grows.

The molar clone of the mole has an anterior, posterior and inferior progress zone. The anterior progress zone produces the deciduous molars in the sequence Dm 4, Dm 3, Dm 2, Dm 1 as it grows forwards. The posterior and inferior progress zones produce the permanent molars and premolars respectively (*Fig. 5.5*).

Each of the three dental clones in the mole is initiating teeth at the same time. By reference to the sequence given at the beginning of this section it can be seen that the incisors develop in the sequence 1, 2, 3, the deciduous molars in the sequence 8, 7, 6, 5, and the permanent molars in the sequence 9, 10, 11. The canine clone has no anterior or posterior progress zones, merely an inferior progress zone.

The clone model has the following circumstantial and experimental support. In all mammals the canine and the first incisor and molar appear to develop at independent times from independently developed regions of dental lamina. The remaining teeth are always initiated in sequence from these three centres. Reconstructions of developing jaws indicate that space is created for the deciduous molars (for example) by interstitial growth which separates the developing deciduous canine from the fourth deciduous molar; presumably due to growth of the relevant progress zones.

The model has been tested by the following experiment (Lumsden, 1979). The primordium of a mouse first molar was dissected from the jaw of a 14-day-old embryo and transferred to the anterior chamber of the eye of another mouse. This tissue is equivalent to that in *Fig. 5.3b*. In support of the clone model, the whole molar dentition developed in the new site. It is deduced from the experiment that all the presumptive molar tooth tissue of the mouse is concentrated around the 14-day-old first molar primordium.

The way in which the clone model can be applied to the development of gradients in tooth shape will be described in the next chapter.

REFERENCES AND FURTHER READING

De Beer G. R. (1947) The differentiation of neural crest cells into visceral cartilages and odontoblasts in ambystoma, and a re-examination of the germ-layer theory. *Proc. R. Soc.* **134-B**, 377.

Bhaskar S. N. (1980) *Orban's Oral Histology and Embryology*. St Louis, Mosby.

Butler P. M. (1939) 1. Studies of the mammalian dentition. Differentiation of the post-canine dentition. *Proc. Zool. Soc. Lond.* **109-B**, 1.

Butler P. M. (1967) Dental merism and tooth development. *J. Dent. Res.* **46**, 845.

Fitzgerald L. R. (1969) Mechanisms controlling morphogenesis in developing teeth. *J. Dent. Res.* **48**, 726.

Gaunt W. A. and Miles A. E. W. (1967) Fundamental aspects of tooth morphogenesis. In: Miles A. E. W. (ed.), *Structural and Chemical Organization of Teeth*, vol. 1. New York, Academic.

Hurmerinta K. and Thesleff I. (1981) Ultrastructure of the epithelial–mesenchymal interface in the mouse tooth germ. *J. Craniofacial Genetics* **1**, 191.

Kollar E. J. and Lumsden A. G. S. (1979) Tooth morphogenesis: the role of the innervation during induction and pattern formation. *J. Biol. Buccale* **7**, 49.

Lumsden A. S. (1979) Pattern formation in the molar dentition of the mouse. *J. Biol. Buccale* **7**, 77.

Ooë T. (1957) On the early development of human dental lamina. *Okajiimas Folia Anat. Jap.* **30**, 197.

Ooë T. (1981) *Human Tooth and Dental Arch Development*. Tokyo, Ishyaku.

Osborn J. W. (1973) The evolution of dentitions. *Am. Scient.* **61**, 548.

Osborn J. W. (1978) Morphogenetic gradients: fields versus clones. In: Butler P. M. and Joysey K. A. (ed.), *Development, Structure and Functions of Teeth* Oxford, Academic, pp. 171–201.

Osman A. and Ruch J. V. (1975) Répartition topographique des mitoses dans les territoires odontogènes de la machoire inférieure de l'embryon de souris. *J. Biol. Buccale* **3**, 117.

Pourtois M. (1961) Contribution à l'étude des bourgeons dentaires chez la souris. I. Périodes d'induction et de morphodifférentiation. *Arch. Biol. Liege* **72**, 17.

Scott J. H. (1967) *Dento-facial Growth and Development*. London, Pergamon.

Tonge C. H. (1953) The early development of teeth. *Proc. R. Soc. Med.* **46**, 313.

CHAPTER 6

MORPHOGENESIS

INTRODUCTION

Morphogenesis is the development of the shape of organs rather than of individual cells. It includes shapes such as gastrulating embryos, the neural tube, tooth germs, bones and whole limbs.

The shape of a protein is determined by its sequence of amino-acids and this sequence is represented by a corresponding sequence of nucleic acids (DNA). The controls which lead to the developing shape of an organ have proved far more difficult to understand. To state that these shapes are genetically determined provides little advance on a theory of divine creation. In essence, all such a statement says is that they are not environmentally determined.

All human lower right first molars look alike and are quite different from those of a cat. The many similarities between the teeth of animals comprising each mammalian species and their differences from the teeth of other mammalian species make it quite obvious that the occlusal morphology of a tooth is to a great extent genetically determined. From a detailed study of molar morphology in identical human twins it has been suggested that the presence and shape of even quite minor cuspules and fissures are probably genetically determined. Were it not for this study it might have been argued that local mechanical differences accounted for all minor variations between teeth. Similar studies have shown that the shape of the shovel-shaped incisor is also genetically determined. But these genetic studies do not reveal the mechanisms operating on the ball of cells comprising a tooth bud inducing it to develop its own unique shape.

An isolated tooth germ at the cap stage of development when cultured *in vitro* changes in shape as it grows. The changes in shape, as opposed to increase in size, are closely linked with cytodifferentiation and histodifferentiation in the absence of which a mere ball of identical cells would be formed. Nearly all attempts to understand morphodifferentiation are based on models which attempt to understand cytodifferentiation because the two seem to be so closely linked. Wolpert (1978) suggested that morphogenesis comprises three different activities: cytodifferentiation, pattern formation and growth. Cytodifferentiation involves the ways in which cells become different from each other and is 'closest' to DNA. It is the result of induction and differentiation, and has become a field of study for molecular biology and biochemistry. Pattern formation describes how different groups of cells differentiate, move, grow, fold and so on to become arranged in a primordial pattern. It is largely investigated by experimental embryologists who seek to understand developmental controls by surgically interfering with embryogenesis. The third feature of morphogenesis, growth, is of two types: early growth during which shape is initiated, and later growth during which the organ largely increases in size but, broadly speaking, maintains the same shape. Examples of early growth are the appearance within a limb bud of the cartilage model of a humerus and the early growth of a tooth germ during which its ultimate shape is mapped out. Later growth involves the increase in size of the cartilage model of the humerus and its replacement by bone, and the laying down of the mineralized tissues in a tooth.

OBSERVATIONS OF TOOTH MORPHOGENESIS

It is convenient largely to restrict the following account to the development of molar teeth.

The stages in cytodifferentiation of the dental organ have been described in Chapter 5. Until the bell stage it is not easy to define significant differences between the primordia of different teeth. But during the bell stage the junction between the dental organ and the dental papilla folds into the shape of the enamel/dentine junction of the final tooth and this is close to the shape of the fully developed crown. The folding of this junction is an example of pattern formation, but it clearly requires growth and only takes place following a degree of cytodifferentiation in the cells of the dental organ. Later growth involves the formation of the enamel. Minor variations, particularly in the form of small cuspules and fissures, are produced due to regional variations in the thickness of enamel deposited on the enamel/dentine junction. Apart from documenting their existence the development of these minor variations in enamel thickness appears not to have been studied. It seems probable that the constriction of the blood supply to ameloblasts in the region of fissures may be related to the thin enamel often present here.

THE FOLDING OF THE ENAMEL ORGAN

At the start of the bell stage of development, mitosis is continuing in each of the cell layers of the dental organ and the stratum indermedium begins to appear. Most of the cell divisions in the dental papilla are confined to its periphery with only a few in its centre. Cells towards the middle of the internal dental epithelium (IDE) are lengthening, closing the cell free gap between them and the papilla, until they are about 40 µm long; they are cuboidal near the cervical loop (*Fig. 15.1*). As the IDE cells lengthen they induce the adjacent papilla cells to lengthen and the latter begin to take on the characteristics of odontoblasts. They are, of course, pre-odontoblasts since they are not yet producing dentine.

The critical stage in pattern formation now begins. The pre-odontoblasts stop dividing. A little later, in the region of the first cusp to appear, the cells of the IDE stop dividing and apparently buckle upwards towards the external dental epithelium (*Fig. 6.1b*). The cells on the flanks of the presumptive cusp continue dividing. Odontoblasts now differentiate and dentine is formed at the tip of the cusp.

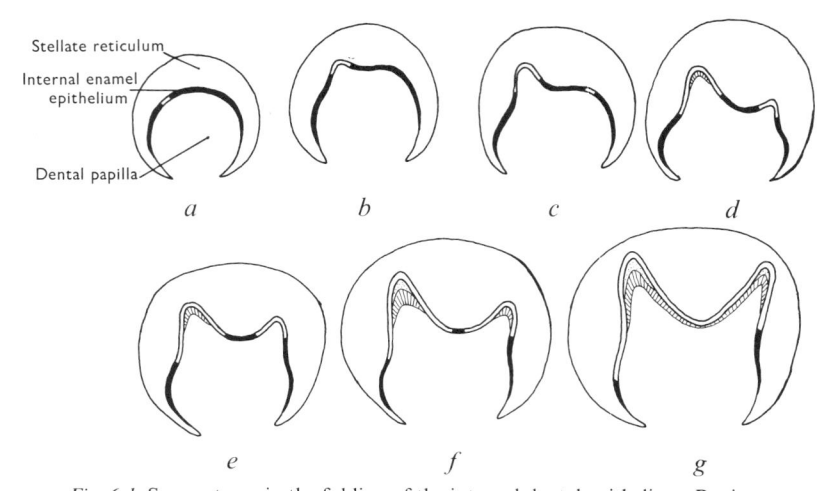

Fig. 6.1. Seven stages in the folding of the internal dental epithelium. Regions in which the cells of the internal dental epithelium are dividing are black; regions in which division has ceased are clear. Enamel is stippled, dentine is cross-hatched. Cusps continue to separate while the cells of the internal dental epithelium are dividing. The final shape of the enamel dentine junction is stabilized when the dentine bridge has connected the two cusps (*g*).

A little later the same sequence of events is repeated in the region of the second presumptive cusp. In a section (*Fig. 6.1d*) the IDE now contains two regions where cells are not dividing, the tips of the presumptive cusps. The IDE cells on the walls of the tooth are still dividing, and those in the valley between the cusps now seem to grow into the papilla, thereby increasing the height of the presumptive cusps in both of which dentine is being formed. The wave of induction and differentiation spreads down into the valley until all the cells have stopped dividing and later a dentine bridge unites the cusps. At the same time similar waves spread down the walls of the tooth.

Cytodifferentiation, pattern formation and growth (cell division) have all been involved in the critical phase at which the IDE/dental papilla interface buckles and the shape of the tooth is moulded.

MINOR PATTERNS

The cusps of teeth are not the smooth symmetrical cones which would be expected to develop from the above description. Even the human canine possesses ridges running from near the cusp tip to the cervical margin of the crown, while close inspection of unworn molars reveals a variety of ridges associated with each cusp, apparently having little or no functional or phylogenetic significance. While many of these features may be accounted for by localized enamel thickenings, those of a more permanent nature, e.g. the oblique ridges of human upper molars, are established at the enamel dentine junction. Investigation into the distribution of dividing cells in developing molars reveals that growth is not even over the entire surface. Indeed, there is often a greater proportion of dividing cells of the inner dental epithelium over one flank of a cusp than another, so that it can be argued that tensional forces are set up which cause the cusp to tilt slightly on the crown. This has been shown in the carnassial teeth of the cat. Until mineralization starts the crown pattern remains pliable and ridges can form, to be stabilized later by the formation of hard dentine and enamel along their crests; there is evidence that apposition of enamel spreads more rapidly along the ridges than over the intervening cuspal surfaces. The ridges so formed serve not only to link the cusps and produce a characteristic crown pattern, but also to provide functional shearing edges. Moreover, the complex of ridges tends to generate intervening fossae into which cusps of the opposing teeth can bite to provide a pestle-and-mortar action.

CONTROLS

There are three levels at which the morphogenesis of the dentition can be studied. The first looks at mechanisms which could control the abrupt differences between the shapes of adjacent teeth (e.g. canine, first premolar) and the gradual differences between a series of teeth (e.g. first, second, third molar). This will be discussed in a later section. The second seeks to find the tissue which controls the shape of an individual tooth (dental organ, dental papilla or another influence). The third looks at the controls exerted at the cellular (e.g. odontoblasts, IDE) or extracellular (e.g. collagen) levels.

TISSUE CONTROL

By immersing dissected lower jaws in trypsin Dryburg (1967) separated oral epithelium from its underlying ectomesenchyme in 9-day-old embryo mice, at which time the mandibular arches have not yet fused in the midline. The epithelium was replaced in such a way that the molar epithelium covered the incisor mesenchyme and the incisor epithelium covered the molar ectomesenchyme. The recombinant was cultured *in vitro*. The tissue did not thrive but the poorly organized rudiments of tooth germs were judged to be molariform where incisor ectomesenchyme was combined with molar epithelium and vice versa. In other words, the dental organ controls shape. Despite efforts by several people, this work, which was reported as an abstract, has so far been found impossible to repeat on such early and fragile embryonic material.

However, a different series of experiments by Kollar and Baird (1970) led to the opposite conclusion. Incisor and molar buds were dissected from the jaws of embryo mice at a rather later stage of development than that used in the previous study. The epithelial and ectomesenchymal parts of the buds were separated; the incisor epithelium was grafted onto the molar ectomesenchyme and the molar epithelium onto the incisor ectomesenchyme. Organ culture of the recombinations revealed that the shape of the resultant tooth was determined by the ectomesenchyme. The ectomesenchyme also possessed the ability to control the activity of embryonic epithelium from many other sites. For example, epithelium which would have developed into skin covering the foot, or into hair follicles, was induced by a molar dental papilla to grow into the dental organ of a molar tooth. These experiments suggest that the ectomesenchyme of a tooth bud determines the shape into which a tooth develops (*see also* Chapter 5).

Although one tissue may indeed have the more important influence, it should be pointed out that neither dental organ nor dental papilla can develop shape alone. Only when together can they produce a recognizable tooth shape.

CELLULAR AND EXTRACELLULAR CONTROL

An increasingly large number of experiments (*in vitro*) have shown that when the synthesis of collagen is inhibited, tooth morphogenesis is prevented. When the inhibitor is removed, morphogenesis begins. Interest centres on the basement membrane and basal lamina between papilla and dental organ. The results are usually interpreted as evidence that collagen, particularly that in the basement membrane, in some way is, or binds, a morphogenetic substance; that collagen carries information which codes for shape. In contrast it can simply be argued that collagen is merely a scaffolding around which shape is built; in the absence of any scaffolding it is impossible to construct and support a complex shape.

It has commonly been shown that morphogenesis cannot proceed without the differentiation of odontoblasts and the internal dental epithelium. This can lead to the interpretation that these cells are the seat of some morphogenetic substance. Alternatively, the elusive morphogenetic factor may be responsible for both differentiation and morphogenesis; the differentiation of cells is not the cause of morphogenesis but both are the result of a third unknown.

The role of cAMP (cyclic adenosine monophosphate) and cGMP (cyclic guanosine monophosphate) has been studied in tissues other than teeth. A very small proportion of the ATP in cells may be broken down by an intracellular enzyme into cAMP. The amount is infinitesimal because about 1000 kg of body tissue may be required to produce 10 µg of cAMP; however, the substance can be synthesized *in vitro* and its activity inhibited *in vivo* in order to facilitate studies of its function(s). It appears that cAMP induces differentiation of cells while cGMP induces cell division and growth. It might therefore be supposed that during growth of the tooth germ the cells of the papilla produce cGMP which is passed into the basement membrane between the dental papilla and the internal dental epithelium. In this position it may become attached to the plasma membranes of the internal dental epithelium, and in some way initiate cell division. At a later stage the papilla will produce less cGMP and more cAMP. This latter substance inhibits cell division and encourages the differentiation of ameloblasts.

MODELS

The identification of a morphogenetic substance or stimulus cannot of itself explain morphogenesis. Changes in shape are brought about through forces produced by the cells which react to the stimulus or stimuli. A model must propose the source(s) of these forces.

The following account is a modification of the model proposed by Butler (1956). The developing tooth germ may be likened to a fluid-filled sphere which is partitioned across the middle by the inner dental epithelium. The stellate reticulum is on one side of the partition and the dental papilla on the other side. The cells of the stellate reticulum are separated from each other by glycosaminoglycans. This substance is intensely hydrophilic and the water which it has absorbed is thought to produce a region of high hydrostatic pressure. On the other side of the partition the growing dental papilla balances this hydrostatic pressure so that the IDE is stabilized between the two. The surrounding dental follicle constricts the tooth germ to an approximately spherical shape. The partitioning sheet of cells (the IDE) increases in surface area by cell division. But its perimeter, the cervical loop, is prevented from expanding by the retaining dental follicle. Evidently, as the surface area of the partition increases it must buckle. By this buckling a primary cuspal elevation of the IDE is produced (*Fig. 6.1*). From a purely mechanistic analogy it might be thought that the IDE could buckle down into the dental papilla rather than up into the stellate reticulum. But the surface of the dental papilla is convex towards the IDE and this will result in any mechanical buckling being towards the stellate reticulum.

It will be recalled that mitosis has ceased at the tip of the cusp but that it is continuing on the flanks. These flanks are now convex towards the dental papilla so that from a purely mechanistic analogy it can be argued that the growing internal dental epithelium would now begin to buckle into the dental papilla. This does in fact occur so that the height of the primary cuspal elevation is increased by a deepening of its flanks down into the dental papilla rather than further growth up into the stellate reticulum (*Fig. 6.1*).

By referring to the above section on the folding of the dental organ, the development of two or more cusps can be understood in terms of the model.

Wessels (1968) has described collagenous filaments which extend from the basement membrane at the periphery of feather primordia into the underlying mesenchyme. He argues that these filaments anchor the surrounding epidermis to the underlying mesenchyme when the feather primordium bulges out onto the surface. A recent histological study (Wigglesworth, personal communication) has identified similar filaments extending from the basement membrane at the depths of fissures into the underlying dental papilla. He proposes these 'anchor fibrils' hold down the presumptive fissure region while the growing pulp pushes up the presumptive cusps.

A very ingenious and compelling model, developed to account for gastrulation, invokes intracellular microfilaments as the source of contractile forces which cause cell layers to buckle (Odell et al., 1981).

Although each of the above models identifies forces which could cause buckling they are incomplete in terms of tooth morphogenesis. They can explain why the IDE buckles but not why it buckles in a specific region. What control specifies the precise locus at which the first cusp of a molar, and each succeeding cusp, develops? Put in another way, what is different between an upper and a lower human first molar? The IDE in each buckles.

There is no satisfactory answer to the above question. Because it opens up the problem of controlling the differences between teeth it is best discussed in the following section.

THE CONTROL OF GRADIENTS IN SHAPE

Merism is the repetition of parts in an organism so as to form a regular pattern. Examples are the limbs of a lobster, the bones in a vertebral column and the teeth in a dentition. It is typical of a meristic series that the basic characteristics of each unit are expressed more strongly in different

MORPHOGENESIS

parts of the series. The problem is what controls the expression of the different characteristics in, for example, a dentition. Cusp number, crown height, root number, mesio-distal dimension and so on are each expressed differently in different regions; the basic plan is the same for all teeth.

A generalized type of model applied to dentitions comes under the heading of 'field theory'. The following brief account is based on an analysis by Osborn (1978).

In field models it is axiomatic that all primordia are identical (e.g. Butler, 1956; Van Valen, 1970). Since they become different they must be operated on by some outside influence. The model continues by implying that all primordia contain the same pattern of targets which code for all possible cusps on a tooth. A field generator situated somewhere in the jaw produces field substances which diffuse through the jaw but are continually being destroyed, with the result that there is a gradient of field substances (*Fig. 6.2*). They are most concentrated at the field generator and most dilute at the furthest distance away from it. According to its concentration a field substance activates target regions in tooth primordia. Because the concentration of field substance is different around each primordium, the targets activated, and therefore the resultant cusps, are

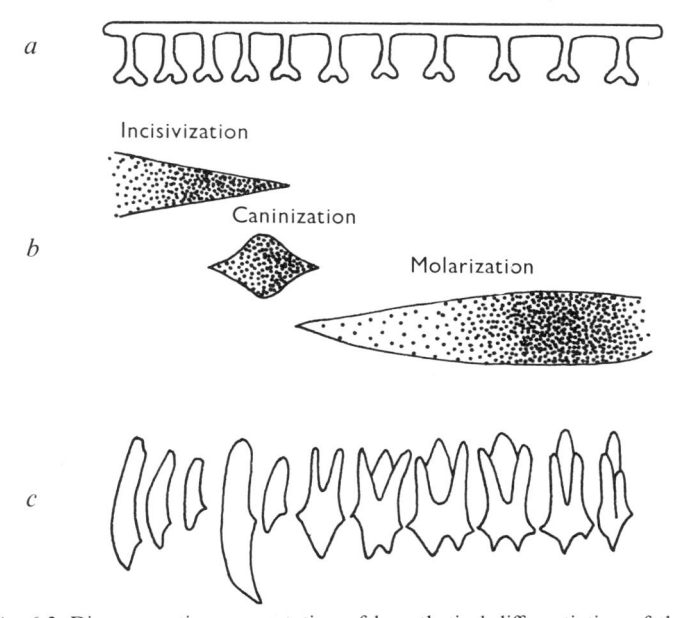

Fig. 6.2. Diagrammatic representation of hypothetical differentiation of the mammalian dentition. *a*, The dental lamina with undifferentiated tooth germs; *b*, Morphogenetic fields believed to influence the development of the tooth germs; *c*, The resulting definitive dentition. (Reproduced from Butler, 1939.)

different. Butler considers that three fields exist (*Fig. 6.2*), each presumably activating different targets (however, note that incisor and molar primordia must all originally possess the same targets if they are identical).

Part of the opposition to the above model poses the question: is it likely that the primordium of a human deciduous incisor developed at 8 weeks in utero is identical to the primordium of the third molar developed at 8 years of age? If they are different the whole foundation of the field model in its application to dentitions is destroyed.

The clone model (*see* Chapter 5) has been applied to the same problem. It has been observed that gradients in the shapes and sizes of teeth seem always to match the sequences in which they develop. The suggestion is made that the shape of a tooth is in some way determined from the moment at which its primordium is initiated. No external influence exists. A gradient in the shapes of teeth develops because, for example, the cells which contribute the second primordium in a sequence have divided more times (they arise from mitoses in the progress zone) than those contributing the first primordium and so on. In support of this view, from the earliest stages at which they can be cultured in isolation from any external influence existing in embryonic jaws (e.g. in the anterior chamber of the eye) tooth germs grow into the shapes they would have developed. Differences between deciduous and permanent molars and premolars, derived from the same (molar) clone, are due to the fact that they develop from anterior, posterior and inferior progress zones respectively.

REFERENCES AND FURTHER READING

Butler P. M. (1956) The ontogeny of molar pattern. *Biol. Rev.* **31**, 30.

Butler P. M. (1979) The ontogeny of mammalian heterodonty. *J. Biol. Buccale* **6**, 217.

Dryburg L. C. (1967) The epigenetics of early tooth development in the mouse. *J. Dent. Res.* **46**, 1264.

Gaunt W. A. (1955) The development of the molar pattern of the mouse. *Acta Anat.* **24**, 249.

Gaunt W. A. (1959) The development of the deciduous cheek teeth of the cat. *Acta Anat.* **38**, 187.

Gaunt W. A. (1961) The development of the molar pattern of the golden hamster. *Acta Anat.* **45**, 219.

Gaunt W. A. and Miles A. E. W. (1967) Fundamental aspects of tooth morphogenesis. In: Miles A. E. W. (ed.), *Structural and Chemical Organization of Teeth*, vol. 1, New York, Academic.

Kollar E. J. (1978) The role of collagen during tooth morphogenesis: some genetic implications. In: Butler P. M. and Joysey K. A. (ed.), *Development, Function and Evolution of Teeth,* New York, Academic, pp. 1–12.

Kollar E. J. and Baird G. R. (1970a) Tissue interactions in embryonic mouse tooth germs. *J. Emb. exp. Morphol.* **24**, 159.

Kollar E. J. and Baird G. R. (1970b) Tissue interactions in embryonic mouse tooth germs. *J. Emb. exp. Morphol.* **24**, 173.

Kraus B. S. and Jordan R. E. (1965) *The Human Dentition before Birth.* London, Kimpton.

Miller W. A. (1969) Inductive changes in early tooth development. 1. A study of mouse tooth development on the chick chorioallantois. *J. Dent. Res.* **48**, 719.

Odell G. M., Oster G., Alberch P. et al. (1981) The mechanical basis of morphogenesis. *Dev. Biol.* **85**, 446.

Osborn J. W. (1978) Morphogenetic gradients: fields versus clones. In: Butler P. M. and Joysey K. A. (ed.), *Development, Function and Evolution of Teeth* New York, Academic, pp. 171–201.

Osborn J. W. (1979) A cladistic interpretation of morphogenesis. *J. Biol. Buccale* **6**, 327.

Slavkin H. C. and Bavetta L. A. (1972) *Developmental Aspects of Oral Biology.* New York, Academic.

van Valen L. (1970) An analysis of developmental fields. *Dev. Biol.* **23**, 456.

Wessels N. K. and Evans J. (1968) The ultrastructure of oriented cells and extracellular materials between developing feathers. *Develop. Biol.* **18**, 42.

Wolpert L. (1978) Pattern formation and the development of the chick limb. *Birth Defects. Original Article Series* **14**, 547.

Wood B. F. and Green L. J. (1968) Second premolar morphologic trait similarities in twins. *J. Dent. Res.* **48**, 74.

CHAPTER 7

GROWTH OF THE TOOTH GERM

The term 'growth' encompasses all the processes involving increase in size and weight of the individual from the time the egg is fertilized. In the two preceding chapters some of the histological changes within the tooth germ from its time of inception have been indicated but little has so far been said concerning the progressive changes in the dimensions of the developing tooth germ. In this dimensional sense growth involves changes not only in absolute size but also in the relative proportions of component parts, both of which determine the definitive form.

Before proceeding further it will be helpful to mention briefly some of the techniques available for measuring growth of tooth germs. It is possible by careful microdissection to free the developing tooth germs from the surrounding tissues and to measure their gross dimensions directly. However, owing to the amount of fluid in the stellate reticulum and the delicate nature of the outer dental epithelium in the early tooth germ, great care is necessary to prevent the dental organ collapsing and causing distortion of the inner dental epithelium. With the onset of dentinogenesis, the dentine caps can be dissected out and stained with alizarin red S which differentially stains mineralized regions on the tooth crown. Alternatively, whole jaws may be stained with alizarin red solution and then rendered transparent to allow direct measurements of the stained dentine caps in situ. The total volumes of enamel and dentine formed can be measured directly from dissected teeth. When mineralized, the dentine and enamel caps become radio-opaque and their dimensions can be measured directly by radiographs *in vivo*.

However, from the two previous chapters it is clear that much of the crown pattern is defined by the soft tissues before mineralization starts, and that the crown form results from developmental interaction between the dental organ and the dental papilla, neither of whose dimensions can be measured accurately except in histological sections. Therefore, in order to study the growth of the very early germ, and especially the relative contribution of the soft tissue components, serial sections of histologically fixed tooth germs have been laboriously analysed. Each technique is suited to investigating a particular developmental stage of the tooth germ, the collected results depicting the overall growth picture.

From what has already been said concerning cusp development it is clear that the distances between developing cusp tips increase as the crown becomes larger (*Fig. 6.1d–f*). It will be recalled that the cusps sometimes tilt during development and this is an additional factor determining intercuspal distance. Once the spreading front of mineralized tissue reaches the floors of the intervening valleys, the flanking dentine cusps are stabilized and their intercuspal distances remain constant (*Fig. 6.1g*). Any further changes in the sharpness of ridges and cusps will then be due to differences in the thickness of enamel secreted on the dentine template.

Consider the two ways in which the length of the internal dental epithelium might increase during development. During the cap stage, all these epithelial cells seem to be capable of dividing and no ameloblasts are being differentiated. This suggests that there would be a continuous increase in the number of dividing cells and therefore that growth would accelerate. But at a later stage growth is confined to the cervical loop, and it might be that for each cell which now divides another differentiates to become an ameloblast. Under these conditions the number of dividing cells would remain constant and growth would be constant rather than accelerating. We could distinguish between these two types of growth by measuring the length of the internal dental epithelium in tooth germs of different ages. If growth is constant, and length is plotted against age, the resultant line would be straight, but if growth accelerates the line would be curved. For the latter case, ideal conditions would lead to a straight line if log length were plotted against time.

Most growth studies reveal an initial acceleration from a slow start, followed by a constant rate of increase ending with a period of deceleration. Consider growth in the mesiodistal diameter of human lower first deciduous molars (*Fig. 7.1*). We can distinguish two parts of this curve; it is straight up till about 22 weeks and then it is curved. Because length (mesiodistal diameter) rather than log length has been plotted against time, we might conclude that from 11 to 22 weeks the number of dividing cells does not significantly increase. In other words, many of the dividing cells are differentiating rather than contributing to an increase in the population of dividing cells.

When both cusps start to mineralize the rate of growth decreases, and when they are joined by dentine across the middle of the tooth (starred in *Fig. 7.1*) the decrease in growth rate becomes more obvious. The apparent absence of an initial acceleration in the growth rate demonstrated by *Fig. 7.1* is probably due to the fact that data for all 11-day-old tooth germs have been pooled. Thus, the measurement at this time (about 0·8 mm) includes tooth germs which may range from 0·2 to 1·2 mm (for instance). It is probably during increase from 0·1 mm to 1·2 mm that growth is accelerating. Closely timed measurements of growing deciduous incisors and canines show the sigmoid curve predicted above (*Fig. 7.2*).

It has been shown for lower deciduous molars that the rate of growth in the mesiodistal diameter exceeds that in the buccolingual diameter. Hence the definitive crown is longer than it is broad. The corresponding upper primary molars grow more rapidly along the buccolingual than the mediodistal diameter and the resultant crown is broader than long (*Fig. 7.3*). Similar results have been obtained from measurements of developing

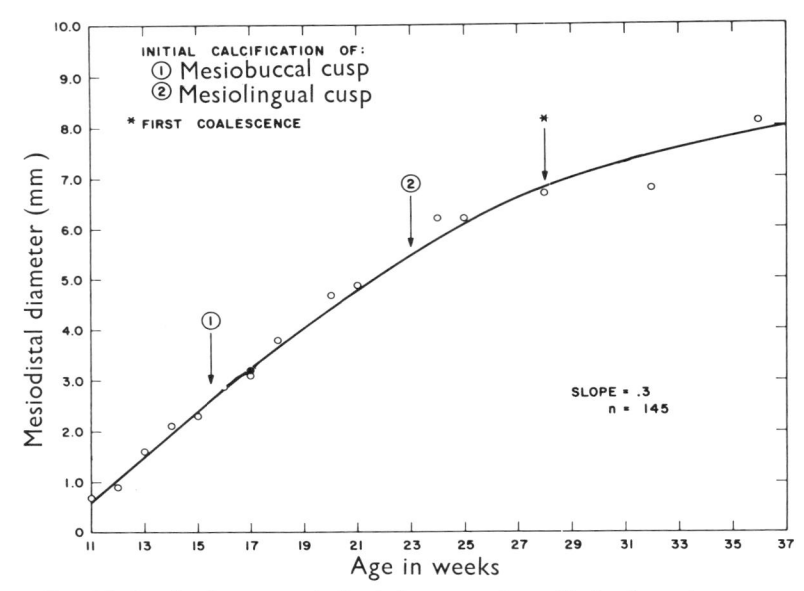

Fig. 7.1. Graph of mean mesiodistal diameters of mandibular first primary molars plotted against age. (*Fig.* reproduced from Kraus and Jordan, 1965.)

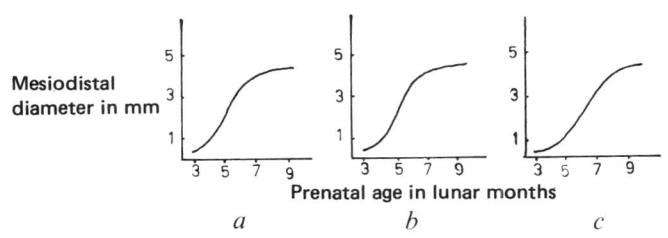

Fig. 7.2. Growth of human (*a*) Di$_1$, (*b*) Di$_2$, and (*c*) Dc. (Data from Oöe T. (1981) *Human Tooth and Dental Arch Development.* Tokyo, Ishiyaku.

mouse molars. These teeth all grow very rapidly by increase in size and number of cells up to the time of completion of the crown pattern which roughly coincides with the appearance of the mineralized tissues. Thereafter, a slower rate of growth continues by accretion of enamel.

Consider, now, growth in height of the tooth. The height of the enamel organ measured along an axis passing vertically through its centre is contributed by the internal dental epithelium, some of whose cells are dividing and some of which have ceased dividing, and by the cuspal enamel together with its associated enamel organ (*Fig. 7.4*). The height of the tooth can be increased by the deposition of cuspal enamel or by an

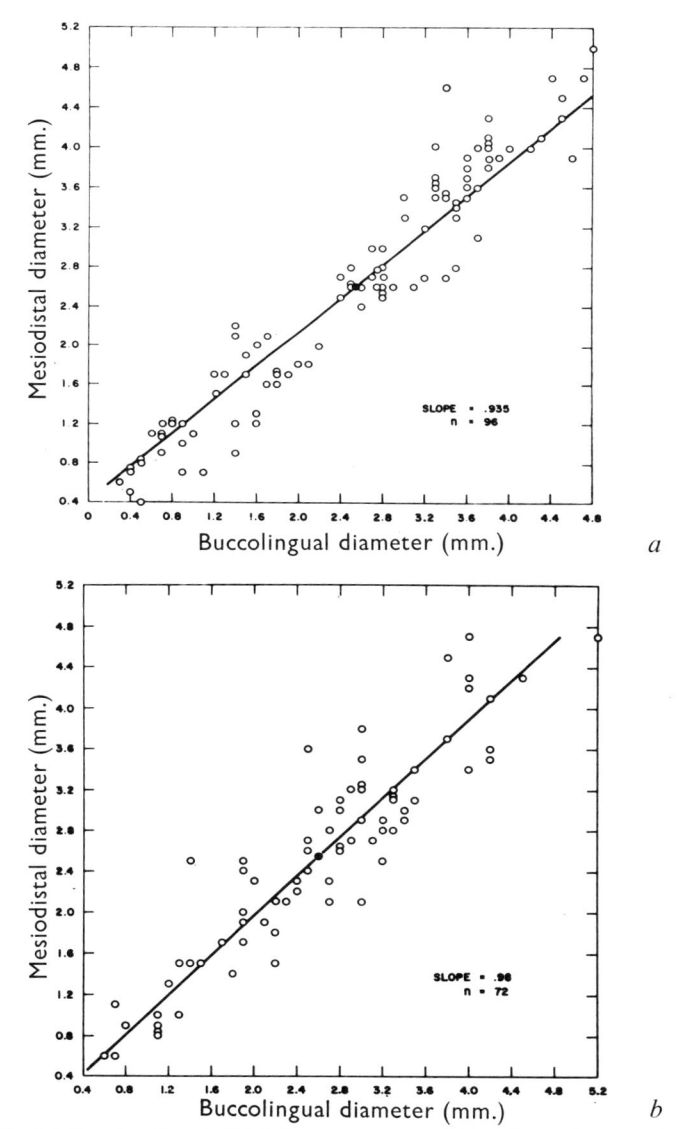

Fig. 7.3. Graphs of mesiodistal diameters of, *a*, maxillary first primary molars and, *b*, maxillary second primary molars, plotted against buccolingual diameters.

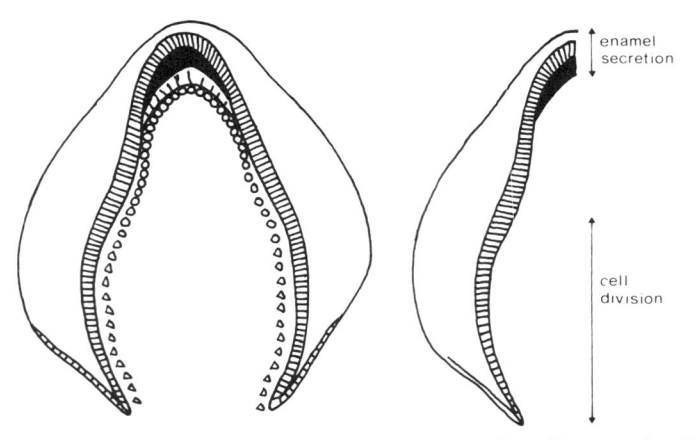

Fig. 7.4. The crown height of a growing tooth is contributed by enamel and by the internal dental epithelium.

increase in the height of the internal dental epithelium (at the cervical loop) due to cell division. Enamel is deposited at the same rate in most human teeth (about 4 µm/day). Therefore *differences* in the rates at which teeth grow in height must be due to *differences* in the rate at which the internal dental epithelium grows in height. This will depend on two factors: the time it takes each cell to divide and the size of the population of dividing cells. It is differences in this latter population which probably account for differences in the rates at which the heights of teeth increase. The size of this population depends on the rate of cell division, and on the rate at which cells are removed from the population by differentiating into ameloblasts (which do not divide). Therefore, if the rate of cell differentiation is slowed down, we might expect the height of the tooth to increase more rapidly because more and more dividing cells are being produced. From measurements of growing deciduous molars and first permanent molars it appears that the increased height of first molars is due to a delay in the times at which cells differentiate.

It is known that the tissue components of the developing mouse molar do not all grow at the same rate. The rate of growth of the surface area of the inner dental epithelium is most rapid up to the time of completion of the definitive shape of the presumptive enamel–dentine junction. During this time, mitosis figures are abundant in the inner dental epithelium particularly in the presumptive cingulum zone, and growth consists essentially of cell multiplication. This is the time when the inner dental epithelium is functioning as a surface of metabolic exchange between the dental organ and the papilla and coincides with a maximum vascular supply to the papilla. Although little corresponding evidence is yet available for the human developing tooth, occasional references are encountered in the literature showing a similar pattern of distribution of mitosis figures, so that it is reasonable to suppose the growth processes in the different teeth to be closely comparable (*Fig. 7.5*). In the mouse molars the dental organ has a slightly greater volume than the dental papilla up to the time the crown pattern is completed, though both components grow at the same rate. Later, however, as the stellate reticulum becomes reduced, the dental organ shrinks, becoming smaller than the dental papilla. Descriptive accounts, as opposed to actual measurements, suggest that the dental organ grows rapidly in a basal direction to enshroud the papilla, but in the mouse at least it is known that this apparent enshrouding is in reality due to an overall change in shape of the inner dental epithelium from hemispherical to conical.

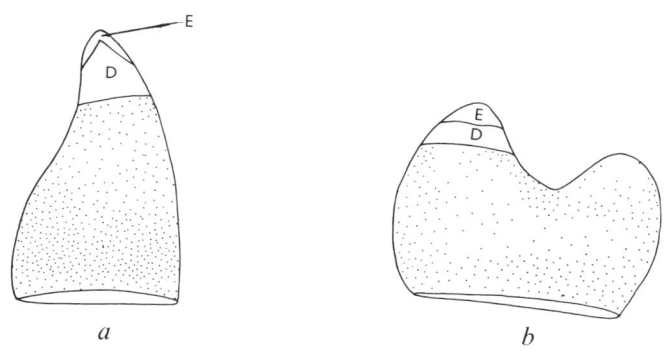

Fig. 7.5. Distribution of dividing cells in the inner dental epithelium of human tooth germs. *a*, Note the greater density of dividing cells in the cingulum zone. *b*, Note area of dividing cells between the cusps. Not to scale. D, dentine; E, enamel.

This suggests that descriptive accounts of developing human teeth need to be checked by actual measurements of the component tissues of the developing tooth.

In general terms, then, the present state of our knowledge enables us to say that growth of the tooth germ comprises two phases. During the first (soft tissue) phase the dental organ rapidly changes in both size and shape. Cells are rapidly dividing and morphogenetic processes are taking place. In the succeeding (hard tissue) phase the shape has already been established and there is only growth in size due to the deposition of enamel and dentine. The rate of cell division is waning and hard tissues are being deposited.

REFERENCES AND FURTHER READING

Butler P. M. (1968) Growth of the human second lower deciduous molar. *Arch. Oral Biol.* **13**, 671.

Butler P. M. (1971) In: Dahlberg A. A. (ed.), *Dental Morphology and Evolution*. Chicago, University of Chicago Press, p. 3.

Christensen G. J. (1967) Occlusal morphology of human molar tooth buds. *Arch. Oral Biol.* **12**, 141.

Gaunt W. A. (1963) An analysis of the growth of the cheek teeth of the mouse. *Acta Anat.* **54**, 220.

Kraus B. S. and Jordan R. E. (1965). *The Human Dentition before Birth*. London, Kimpton.

Ooë T. (1981) *Human Tooth and Dental Arch Development*. Tokyo Ishiyaku.

Stack M. V. (1964) A gravimetric study of crown growth rate of the human deciduous dentition. *Biol. Neonat.* **6**, 197.

Turner E. P. (1963) Crown development in human deciduous molar teeth. *Arch. Oral Biol.* **8**, 523.

CHAPTER 8

THE BLOOD SUPPLY TO THE TEETH

In studying the vascular supply to the dental tissues, it is necessary to determine the origin of the vessels, their arrangement, distribution and density both within and around the tooth. Where tissue development is rapid there is a rich blood supply, and the more complex the organization of the particular structure, whether anatomically or physiologically, the more abundant are the anastomoses of blood capillaries to be found. Density of the capillary network is most important in controlling the growth of the tissue, for on it depends the hypertrophy or atrophy of the tissue supplied. Abnormal blood supply leads to hypertrophy or atrophy of the whole or parts of the tooth, irregularities of surface configuration, defects in quality of the organic or inorganic components, and other structural or physiological deviations from the typical form.

Although it is possible by laborious analysis of serial sections to reconstruct a panoramic view of vascular distribution to the teeth, the majority of investigations so far reported are based upon procedures involving the replacement of the blood in the vessels by an injected mass whose properties determine the techniques of examination subsequently employed. Coloured dyes, india ink, tinted latex or coloured precipitates formed within the vessels by interaction between injected chemicals, all reveal the vascular architecture with great clarity, especially when combined with bulk clearing of the specimens, rendering them transparent. In recent years acid corrosion techniques have been developed. The surrounding tissues are removed by a corrosive fluid, leaving a three-dimensional model of the vascular system. Radio-opaque injection media enable the vascular pattern to be studied radiographically. Two new techniques have recently proved useful in studies of vascular distribution. One technique involves the use of plastic microspheres of known dimension which are injected directly into an artery and allowed to circulate. The microspheres lodge in that portion of the vascular bed where the vessels are of the same diameter as the microspheres. When histological sections are examined the plastic microspheres are clearly seen marking the vessels in which they have lodged. In this way the distribution of any selected part of the arterial system can be studied. The second technique is the histochemical demonstration of adenosine triphosphatase (ATP-ase) in blood vessel walls.

Two basic difficulties are common to all injection techniques. First, the substance must be injected into fresh material under sufficient pressure to fill completely the vascular system but not so great as to rupture the vessels. This gives a picture of the entire vacular bed. However, the entire vascular bed is not fully patent at any one time during life; the pressure applied at the time of injection must certainly have opened a proportion of the smaller channels which would normally be temporarily collapsed. The second problem arises from the technical difficulty of representing a three-dimensional system on a two-dimensional picture. Though absence of the third dimension in the illustrations can be compensated for by written description, the entire complexity of the injected system can only be seen in the original model.

The few published accounts concerning blood supply to primate and human dentitions are in broad agreement with the much more detailed investigations relating to the corresponding system in small mammals. Hence, the picture of vascular supply to the teeth presented in the following paragraphs will be a composite one.

The mammalian upper teeth and their supporting tissues all derive their blood supply from branches of the superior dental arteries, supplemented to varying degrees by branches of the palatal vessels. The corresponding lower teeth and their supporting structures are supplied by branches of the inferior dental arteries which lie within the inferior dental canals; additional supply is derived from branches of the lingual vessels. As stated in Chapter 4, these vessels are present in the jaws of very early cat embryos, even before the appearance of tooth germs. From these as yet thin-walled vessels capillaries arise which are concentrated along the jaws in localized regions which indicate the sites of future tooth germs. In the regions between the future tooth germs, and also in the rodent diastema, there is a sharp reduction in the capillary concentration. Such vascular arrangements have not been reported in primate or human fetal jaws, though it is very probable that here too a closely comparable situation could be demonstrated.

Reconstructions of mammalian and primate tooth germs from serial sections show that groups of blood vessels, originating from the superior and inferior dental arteries, first pass into the dental papilla at the cap stage of development. Detailed analysis of these vessels in the mouse molars (*Fig. 8.1*) shows that they increase in number during the period of histo-differentiation of the tooth germ, reaching a maximum concentration immediately before the phase of most active folding of the inner dental epithelium. Gradually, with the onset of dentinogenesis, the number of vessels decreases and then becomes stabilized for that particular tooth. It will also be seen from *Fig. 8.1* that the total blood flow, computed from the mean diameters of the vessels, increases in parallel manner during this vital morphogenetic period.

At no time during development do blood vessels penetrate into the dental organ, so that up to the start of dentinogenesis the inner dental epithelium probably obtains the majority of its nutrient via the papillary vessels rather than via the outer dental epithelium.

It would thus appear that when dentine is produced it forms a barrier

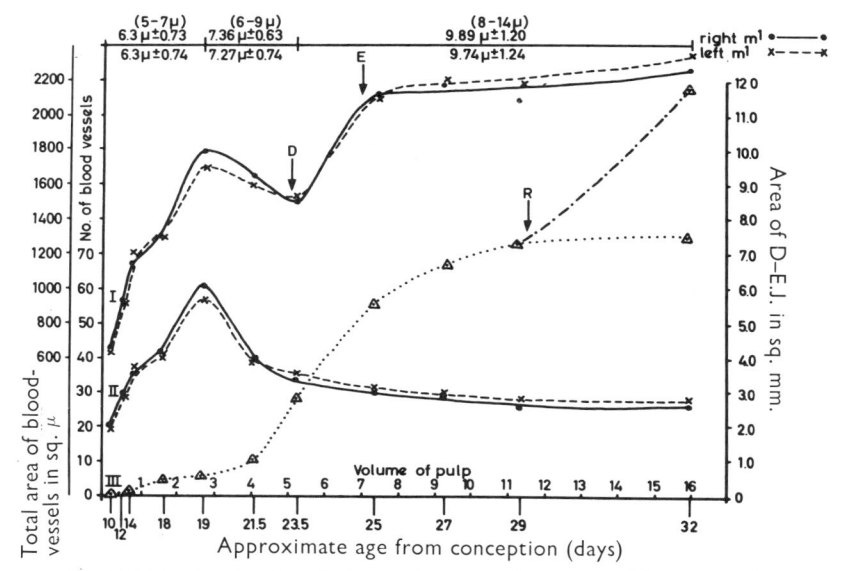

Fig. 8.1. Graphs showing: I, the total cross-sectional area of blood vessels entering the base of the dental papilla in the upper first mouse molar; II, the numbers of such vessels; III, the area of the enamel–dentine junction, all plotted against age. D, Time of start of dentinogenesis; E, time of start of amelogenesis; R, onset of root formation. The mean diameters of the vessels are shown. (*Figs. 8.1* and *8.2* modified from Gaunt, 1960.)

which prevents further metabolic exchange between the dental organ and the dental papilla. This suggestion has received support from histochemical evidence and from the cytological rearrangement of the organelles within the cells of the inner dental epithelium (*see* Chapter 15). Lying adjacent to the outer dental epithelium is a plexus of blood vessels which originate partly from the basal vessels before they pass into the dental papilla, and partly from the periosteal plexus associated with the developing tooth socket.

The blood vessels passing into the dental papilla branch successively, their finest terminations pushing between the odontoblasts as capillary loops from a sub-odontoblastic plexus.

Before the roots are formed, the vessels entering the papilla congregate in groups whose number and position coincide with the number and location of the roots specific to that tooth (*Fig 8.2*). It has been suggested that each of these vascular bundles supplies a separate growth centre within the papilla, though so far without conclusive evidence. As the tooth ages so the pulp chamber diminishes in volume (*see* Chapter 23), the apical foramen becomes progressively narrowed by invading cement and the blood supply becomes reduced. Thus it is that the tooth in old age receives

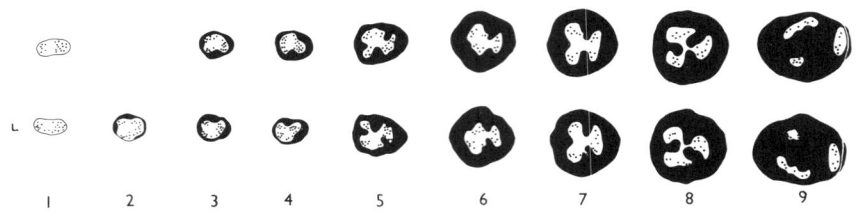

Fig. 8.2. Apical views of the developing left and right second upper molar of the mouse showing the blood vessels entering the dental papilla. Each dot represents a blood vessel.

but a very small proportion of its original blood supply and the viability of the pulp diminishes.

The blood supply to the tissues surrounding the tooth which include the periodontal ligament, the gingiva, the alveolar bone and the epithelial attachment must now be considered.

Examination of material, utilizing the techniques already described, reveals an astonishing vascular density in the tissues adjacent to the tooth. The main supply to the ligament is via the dental artery (*Fig.* 8.3). This artery initially has an intrabony course and gives off alveolar branches.

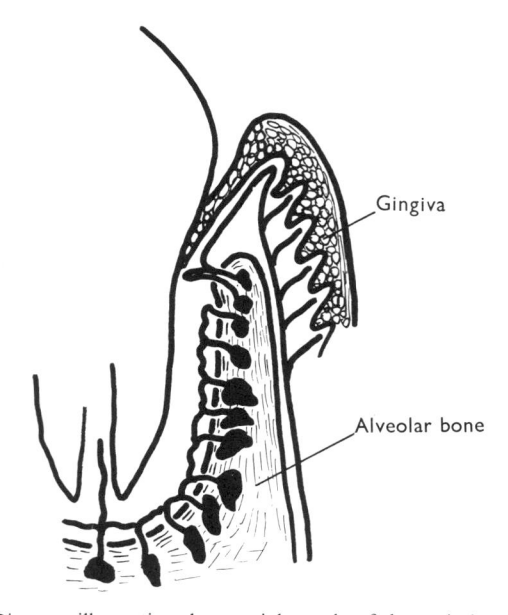

Fig. 8.3. Diagram illustrating the arterial supply of the periodontium.

THE BLOOD SUPPLY TO THE TEETH

One enters the periodontium apically, gives off two longitudinal periodontal arteries and then continues to supply the pulp. Interalveolar arteries ascend to the crest of the alveolus giving off many perforating branches which enter the periodontal ligament at right angles to the socket wall. At the crest of the alveolus these vessels continue on to supply the attachment epithelium and the col area. The perforating arteries are numerous and have been shown to increase in number from tooth to tooth towards the posterior teeth and, in single-rooted teeth, to be greatest in number in the gingival third of the ligament and least in the middle third. The perforating arteries run parallel to the fibre bundles of the ligament and form an arcading network closer to the bone surface than to the cement surface. The classic description of longitudinal arteries running in the periodontal ligament has been questioned. When plastic microspheres are injected into the arterial system they are only found lodged in the perforating arteries. This means that either the longitudinal vessels described after injection techniques represent the venous return or they are of such a diameter that the plastic microspheres do not lodge within their lumen. In view of the profuse arterial supply via the socket wall it is more than likely that the longitudinal vessels are associated with the venous drainage of the ligament.

The blood supply to the gingiva and attachment apparatus shows distinct regional differences. The marginal and attached gingiva receive blood from vessels running in the periosteum of the alveolar process. Branches from these vessels run perpendicular to the surface and form loops within the connective tissue papillae of the gingiva. The vessels supplying the crevicular and attachment epithelium, however, show a different disposition. These are derived mainly from intrabony arteries which leave the alveolar process in the crestal area and pursue a course close to and parallel with the epithelium forming a rich network of vessels. In the region of the col, vessels leave the crest of the alveolar bone and run perpendicularly to the surface of the col. Close to the surface they bend sharply and run parallel to the basement membrane supporting the col epithelium. The difference in the spatial arrangement of vessels in the attached gingiva and the crevicular epithelium most likely reflects the differences in the architecture of the junction between epithelium and its supporting connective tissue. In the presence of inflammation the flat junction supporting the crevicular and attachment epithelium changes and pegs of proliferative epithelium are found. At the same time the vascular supply to this region now develops looped vessels.

Thus essentially the blood supply to the periodontium can be divided into three zones: that to the periodontal ligament, that to the gingiva facing the oral cavity, and that to the gingiva facing the tooth. However, anastomoses have been demonstrated between all three areas and this allows for a considerable collateral circulation in the supporting tissues of the tooth.

REFERENCES AND FURTHER READING

Birn H. (1966) The vascular supply of the periodontal membrane. *J. Periodont. Res.* **1**, 51.

Egelberg J. (1966) The blood vessels of the dentino-gingival junction. *J. Periodont. Res.* **1**, 163.

Folke L. E. A. and Stallard R. E. (1967) Periodontal microcirculation as revealed by plastic microspheres. *J. Periodont. Res.* **2**, 53.

Gaunt W. A. (1960) The vascular suuply in relation to the formation of roots on the cheek teeth of the mouse. *Acta Anat.* **43**, 116.

Kindlova M. (1965) The blood supply of the marginal periodontium in *Macacus rhesus. Arch. Oral Biol.* **10**, 869.

CHAPTER 9

COLLAGEN

Collagen is an essential constituent of connective tissue which means that, apart from enamel, it is found in all dental tissue. Because collagen is a major component of bone, dentine, cement and periodontal ligament, and as it has been suggested that it might be necessary for the initiation of mineralization and that it might provide the force for tooth eruption, it is evident that a working knowledge of this fibrous protein is necessary for students of dental histology.

THE COLLAGEN MOLECULE

When connective tissue is examined with the electron microscope, collagen fibrils can be readily identified because of characteristic repetitive cross-banding of the fibril occurring at every 64 nm. Each fibril is made up of many individual collagen molecules held together in an exact manner by a series of intermolecular chemical linkages. Each collagen molecule is long (280 nm) and thin (1·35 nm) and consists of three polypeptide chains, each containing about 1000 amino-acids. Each polypeptide chain is wound in a left-handed helix and, to form the classic triple helix of the collagen molecule, the three chains are coiled around each other in a slower right-handed 'super-helix' which is stabilized by inter-chain hydrogen bonds.

Not only does the collagen molecule have this distinctive structure but it also has a distinctive chemical composition. Of the 20 amino-acids found in collagen 4 (glycine, alanine, proline and hydroxyproline) make up two-thirds of the molecule. The amino-acid hydroxylysine is characteristic of collagen and has not so far been found in other tissue proteins. Hydroxyproline is found predominantly in collagen but also occurs in small amounts in elastin.

Collagen contains glucose and galactose (typically less than 1 per cent by weight) and is therefore technically a glycoprotein.

In recent years it has become apparent that there are several genetically distinct collagen molecules. These designated types I–V are the best characterized but there is evidence for others which await detailed study. Type I collagen is the only type found so far in the mineralized connective tissues and predominates in skin, tendon, ligament, etc.; type II collagen is found in cartilage; type III is found together with larger amounts of type I collagen in several soft connective tissues; type IV is the major collagen type in basement membrane, while type V is a minor component in many tissues apparently in association with cell surfaces and basement membranes.

COLLAGEN SYNTHESIS

Collagen is synthesized by the fibroblast (also by the bone, dentine and cement-forming cells) in the following way. The individual polypeptide chains are assembled from the appropriate amino-acids on the rough endoplasmic reticulum. These chains are about 50 per cent longer than those in the final molecule having additional sequences of amino-acids at each end. Certain of the proline and lysine residues within the polypeptide chains are then hydroxylated by the enzymes prolyl hydroxylase and lysyl hydroxylase, respectively, to form hydroxyproline and hydroxylysine. Once hydroxylated, the three polypeptide chains assemble into the triple-helix configuration within the cisternae of the rough endoplasmic reticulum. The molecule, now called procollagen, is transported via transport vesicles to the Golgi apparatus where the molecule is glycosylated. From the secretory surface of the Golgi apparatus vesicles containing the procollagen molecules migrate to the cell surface and discharge their contents into the extracellular environment. As the procollagen is secreted across the cell membrane the terminal peptides are cleaved off by the action of procollagen peptidase and the molecule is now called collagen. The formation and secretion of the collagen molecule takes about 35 minutes and this rate, known as the transit time, together with the intracellular pathway, was determined in part by studying collagen formation in the polarized dentine-forming cell, the odontoblast, using the techniques of autoradiography, immunohistochemistry and electron microscopy. Some recent evidence indicates that the fibroblast and the odontoblast may synthesize more polypeptide chains than are required to form the collagen molecules and that these excess chains are destroyed in the cell. Because this is so it is important to recognize that some older studies concerning the rates of collagen *fibril* formation will have to be reevaluated.

FIBRILLOGENESIS

So far only the synthesis of the collagen molecule has been described. Although a large molecule (about 285 000 daltons) this cannot be seen as a structural entity until sufficient collagen molecules have aggregated together to form a collagen *fibril* which is characterized in the electron microscope by its well-known cross-banding pattern. The term 'collagen *fibre*' indicates an aggregation of sufficient fibrils to be visible with the light microscope. The assembly of collagen molecules into fibrils is generally considered to be an extracellular event and is known as fibrillogenesis.

The mechanism whereby the collagen macromolecules are aggregated is not completely understood but it probably first involves electrostatic forces between charged groups of neighbouring collagen molecules. The evidence for this is as follows. Normal collagen fibrils when viewed with the electron microscope show a characteristic banding with a periodicity of 64 nm. If a solution of collagen molecules is reconstituted in sodium chloride at physiological ionic strength fibrils with the same periodicity are formed. If the concentration of the electrolyte is altered in a specific way collagen fibrils with a repeating band every 280 nm are produced. This effect of the electrolyte environment on the aggregation of collagen molecules is consistent with the presence of electrostatic forces between molecules. Thus the young collagen fibril consists of collagen molecules formed by a triple helix of polypeptide chains joined together by *intra* molecular hydrogen bonds which in turn are aggregated with similar units by means of *inter* molecular electrostatic bonds. It is known that collagen becomes progressively more stable and insoluble as it matures. This maturation involves the development of additional cross-links in the form of covalent bonds between the individual collagen macromolecules. These are believed to be relatively few in number but make a very important contribution to the stability of the fibrils.

The way in which the collagen molecules are packed together to give the collagen fibril with its characteristic 64 nm banding is not yet completely understood. It is known, however, that the molecules are lined up parallel to one another and staggered in the long axis relative to one another by some multiple of the 64 nm periodicity, often called 'D'. Since the molecular length is actually 4·4D this gives rise to a regular series of 'gaps' within the fibrils. The nature and size of the spaces within the collagen fibril are a matter of some importance for, as will be discussed in Chapter 10, it is here that much of the mineral is located in the hard connective tissues such as bone, dentine and cement. Thus, although there are still some points of contention, there is general agreement on the principles involved in collagen synthesis and fibrillogenesis.

COLLAGEN DEGRADATION

So far we have discussed only the synthesis of collagen and its assembly into fibrils. On the basis of biochemical studies it has been appreciated for some time that connective tissue is capable of remodelling and turning over, albeit at different rates in different locations. The implication here is that in a connective tissue which is turning over collagen fibrils must be both synthesized and degraded with the rate for each process being the same if the normal architecture of the tissue is to be preserved. Degradation of collagen has been extensively studied, largely in nonphysiological situations such as inflammation, and it is clear that here the sequence of events is an extracellular breakdown of collagen involving a highly specific enzyme, collagenase, which cleaves the collagen molecule three-quarters of the way along its length with other, less specific, enzymes continuing its degradation.

As collagen constitutes 25 per cent of the body's total protein an indiscriminate release of collagenase would have serious consequences for the well-being of the organism. Several control mechanisms are possible. Thus there is evidence that the enzyme exists in an inactive precursor form and must be activated by other enzymes. Also, it seems that collagenase activity is readily inhibited by some of the normal components of serum, especially the $\alpha 2$ macroglobulin. All the above, though, are extracellular events and it is difficult to equate this extracellular sequence, which might be thought to be somewhat haphazard and non-selective, with the orderly breakdown of collagen which must be needed to maintain architecture in connective tissue as it turns over. It happens that the periodontal ligament is, so far, the connective tissue with the highest known rate of turnover (in the mouse periodontal ligament the half-life of collagen is about 24 hours!) and it has been demonstrated that ligament fibroblasts, as well as synthesizing collagen, also degrade it by phagocytosis and intracellular digestion. The fibroblast can ingest either a single collagen fibril or a group of collagen fibrils so that they come to be inside the cell in a vesicle described as a phagosome. Collagenase and perhaps other proteinases may be involved at some point close to the cell surface not yet determined as the cell cleaves off fragments of collagen fibrils of appropriate size for phagocytosis. Lysosomes then fuse with the collagen-containing phagosomes and discharge their enzyme contents to achieve the final degradation of the collagen molecule in this intracellular location.

The concept of connective tissue turnover and remodelling as achieved by the simultaneous synthesis and degradation of collagen by the fibroblast is an important one (*Fig. 9.1*). It follows that any change in either rate of synthesis or degradation of collagen by the cell will lead to significant changes in connective tissue architecture. For example, vitamin C deficiency interferes with collagen formation by preventing the hydroxylation of proline and lysine, but does not interfere with collagen breakdown. Thus, in the periodontal ligament, if collagen synthesis were to be reduced by a deficiency of vitamin C, and cellular degradation continued, collagen would be lost. This occurs and represents direct evidence for a change in fibroblast function being a cause of connective tissue loss.

Although much of the work characterizing cellular involvement in collagen degradation was undertaken studying the periodontal ligament (because of its high rate of turnover), evidence is rapidly accumulating that this ability is a property of other soft connective tissue fibroblasts,

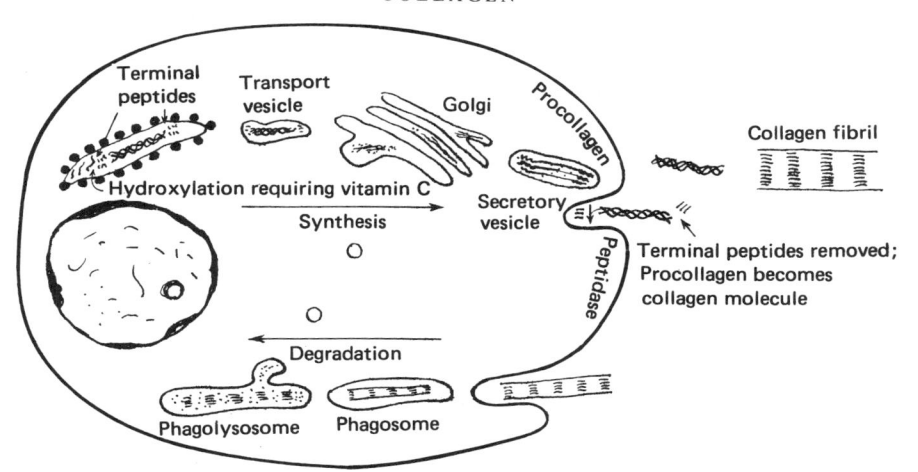

Fig. 9.1. Diagram summarizing the synthetic and degradative functions of the fibroblast.

given the appropriate circumstances. Thus, collagen phagocytosis has been described in healing skin wounds, in scar tissue, in the fibrogenetic phase of fracture repair and in a number of connective tissue lesions.

Enough has now been written for an appreciation of how fairly small variations in collagen structure and fibroblast function permit a number of permutations which may markedly affect the character of any connective tissue. The amount and deposition of the collagen fibre bundles are variable factors and on this basis loose, dense, regular and irregular connective tissue are recognized. Then the number and type of cross-linkage may be varied so that we have connective tissue in which the collagen exhibits different degrees of maturity and stability. The rate of collagen turnover may also be varied in different connective tissues and there is evidence that the amount of intramolecular space in collagen may be varied between, for example, hard and soft connective tissue. Finally, there are the genetically distinct collagen types. Clearly many permutations are possible to permit connective tissue to serve its many differing functions in the economy of the organism.

This chapter has dealt with collagen and, as a necessary consequence, the connective tissue cell, the fibroblast. Because collagen is such a major protein, constituting 25 per cent of the body's total protein complement, other functions of the fibroblast unrelated to collagen synthesis and degradation tend to be overlooked. It must not be forgotten that the fibroblast is also responsible for the synthesis and maintenance of the other major component of connective tissue, namely the ground substance which consists of proteoglycans, glycosoaminoglycans, glycoproteins and glycolipids, as well as the other fibrous components found in connective tissue, such as elastin and oxytalin. Also, as we shall see in Chapter 20, an important contractile function for the fibroblast in relation to tooth eruption has been postulated.

REFERENCES AND FURTHER READING

Eastoe J. E. (1971) The structure and behaviour of connective tissues. In: *The Prevention of Periodontal Disease*. London, Kimpton, p. 89.

Eastoe J. E. (1976) Collagen chemistry and tissue organization. In: Poole D. F. G. and Stack M. V. (ed.), *The Eruption and Occlusion of Teeth*. London, Butterworths.

Eisen A. Z. and Gross J. (1965) The role of epithelium and mesenchyme in the production of a collagenolytic enzyme and a hyaluronidase in the anuran tadpole. *Develop. Biol.* **12**, 408.

Grant M. E. and Prockop D. J. (1972) Biosynthesis of collagen. *New Engl. J. Med.* **286**, 194.

Grant R. A., Horne R. W. and Cox R. W. (1965) New model for the tropocollagen macromolecule and its mode of aggregation. *Nature, Lond.* **207**, 822.

Gross J. and Lapiere C. M. (1962) Collagenolytic activity in amphibian tissues: a tissue culture assay. *Proc. Natl Acad. Sci. U.S.A.*, **48**, 1014.

Harris E. D., Jr and Krans S. M. (1974) Collagenase (3 parts). *Med. Progr.* **291**, 557, 605. 652.

Katchburian E. (1973) Membrane-bound bodies as initiators of mineralization in dentine. *J. Anat.* **116**. 285.

Nylen M. U. and Scott D. B. (1960) Basic studies in calcification. *J. Dent. Med.* **15**, 80.

Ramachandran G. N. (1967) Structure of collagen at the molecular level. In: Ramachandran G. N. (ed.) *Treatise on Collagen. I. Chemistry of Collagen*. New York, Academic, p. 103.

Ross R. (1968) The connective tissue fiber forming cell. In: Gould B. S. (ed.), *Treatise of Collagen*, vol. 2. New York, Academic, p. 1.

Schmitt F. O. and Hodge A. J. (1960) The tropocollagen macromolecule and its properties of ordered interaction. *J. Soc. Leath. Trades Chem.* **44**, 217.

Smith J. W. (1965) Packing arrangement of tropocollagen molecules. *Nature, Lond.* **205**, 356.

Ten Cate, A. R. (1972) Morphological studies of fibrocytes in connective tissue undergoing rapid remodelling. *J. Anat.* **112**, 401.

Ten Cate A. R. and Deporter D. A. (1975) The degradative role of the fibroblast in the remodelling and turnover of collagen in soft connective tissue. *Anat. Rec.* **182**, 1.

Ten Cate A. R. and Freeman E. (1974) Collagen remodelling by fibroblasts in wound repair. Preliminary observations. *Anat. Rec.* **179**, 543.

Ten Cate A. R. and Syrbu S. (1974) A relationship between alkaline phosphatase activity and the phagocytosis and degradation of collagen by the fibroblast. *J. Anat.* **117**, 351.

Weinstock M. and Leblond C. P. (1974) Formation of collagen. *Fed. Proc.* **33**(5), 1205.

Weinstock M. and Leblond C. P. (1974) Synthesis migration and release of precursor collagen by odontoblasts as visualized by radioautography after [^{3}H] proline administration. *J. Cell Biol.* **60**, 92.

CHAPTER 10

HARD TISSUE GENESIS

Most accounts of hard tissue genesis deal specifically with a particular hard tissue and such accounts will also be found later in this book. The purpose of this chapter is to outline the factors common to the formation of all hard tissues, even though the details of structure and composition may differ considerably.

When different forming hard tissues are studied it is readily apparent that there are many common features and these are represented in diagrammatic form in *Fig. 10.1*. Reference to this figure reveals that, in simple terms, hard tissue genesis involves the production of an organic matrix and the introduction into this matrix of mineral salts. The first step, therefore, in producing any hard tissue is to elaborate the organic matrix and for this a specialized cell is required. Such cells differentiate in areas of marked vascularity and have features characteristic of cells actively involved in synthesis and secretion which include large amounts of rough endoplasmic reticulum, many mitochondria, an extensive Golgi complex and the presence of many secretory vesicles.

The organic material secreted by these cells for all the hard tissues, except enamel, consists of collagen molecules aggregated as collagen fibrils and a ground or cementing substance consisting of varying amounts of glycosaminoglycans, glycoproteins and glycolipids. The organic material secreted by the enamel-forming cell is especially distinctive and is not aggregated into a fibrous form, but even so this matrix, as those of the other hard tissues, is capable of accommodating inorganic salts, thereby forming a mineralized tissue.

MINERALIZATION

The mineral in hard tissues consists of calcium and phosphate deposits in the form of calcium hydroxyapatite and amorphous calcium triphosphate. The manner in which they are deposited into an organic matrix is controversial and the subject of continuing study. As there is some uncertainty about the mineralization process, it should be recognized that the description which follows involves some speculation but this is warranted in a text such as this where general principles are being stated. These generalities concern (1) the transport of mineral salts, (2) the initial mineralization of an organic matrix, (3) the continued mineralization of matrix (4) the function of an enzyme, alkaline phosphatase, which may be associated with all facets of hard tissue formation and finally (5) the location of apatite crystals in the organic matrix. Each is discussed in turn.

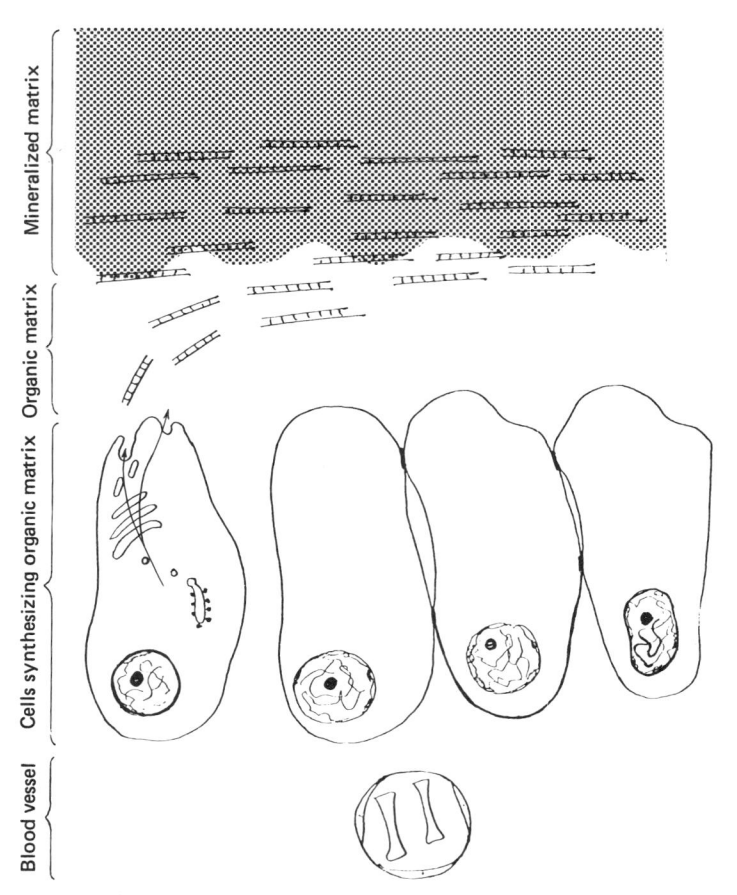

Fig. 10.1. Diagram showing the essential features of hard tissue formation.

The Transport of Mineral Salts

Inorganic salts are brought to the mineralization site via the vascular system and the tissue fluid until the cells associated with the formation of hard tissue are reached. Every mineralization site is, in essence, surrounded by a barrier of cells and this means that inorganic ions must pass either through the cells or between them to reach the organic matrix (*Fig. 10.2*). Here the assumption is made that mineral passes through cells rather than between them because of evidence that mitochondria are involved in the mineralization, that in some instances junctions exist between the cells which will not permit the passage of ions (*see Fig. 2.3*)

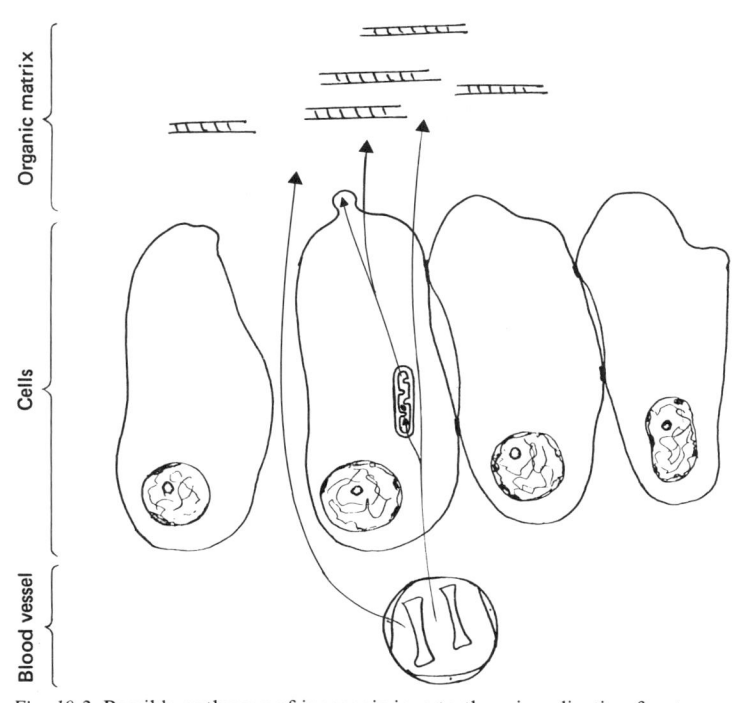

Fig. 10.2. Possible pathways of inorganic ions to the mineralization front.

and, finally, some circumstantial evidence associated with the location of alkaline phosphatase activity during enamel formation.

To reach a cell's interior inorganic salts must, obviously, pass across its plasma membrane and there is a great deal of evidence that alkaline phosphatase activity is required for this transfer. At all locations where it can be predicted that inorganic ions must pass across a cell membrane in any quantity, alkaline phosphatase activity can also be demonstrated. Once within the cell calcium may be stored within its mitochondria. For example, in osteoblasts forming bone and chondrocytes associated with calcifying cartilage a mitochondrial accumulation of inorganic granules, almost certainly amorphous calcium phosphate, can be demonstrated before the onset of mineralization and disappears as mineralization begins in the extracellular compartment.

Initial Mineralization

The inorganic salts now reach the matrix which, in connective tissue, consists of collagen and ground substance pervaded by tissue fluid. In such an environment apatite crystals cannot precipitate spontaneously and for this to occur either there must be a local increase of inorganic ions to permit spontaneous crystal precipitation (homogeneous nucleation) or a nucleating substance must exist to bring about crystallization without the necessity for an increased ionic concentration of mineral (heterogeneous nucleation). Once the first crystal has formed, however, a supersaturated tissue fluid permits the continued deposition of mineral on that crystal. Thus evidence must be sought to demonstrate that one or both mechanisms exist in connective tissue about to mineralize. It is now clear that a cellular mechanism is involved in some instances. Those cells associated with the formation of the matrix of cartilage, woven bone and first-formed (mantle) dentine bud off small membrane-bound vesicles about 0·1 µm in diameter which become lodged between the collagen fibrils of the matrix. Within these vesicles the first apatite crystallites are seen as thin needles at first confined within the vesicle but which grow rapidly and rupture the vesicular membranes to form a cluster of apatite crystals. Such a cluster soon fuses with other clusters formed from adjacent vesicles to create a mineralized matrix. The chemistry of *matrix vesicles* has been extensively studied and alkaline phosphatase activity has been demonstrated in association with them, as has activity of ATPase and the presence of calcium binding lipids all reflecting, in terms of our present state of knowledge, the creation of a localized environment within the vesicle suitable for the initiation of mineralization (*Fig. 10.3*). The concept of the matrix vesicle has recently been challenged on the basis that when sections are prepared in such a way that they never come into contact with any solution no apatite crystallites can be demonstrated in the residues.

Continued Mineralization

It has been pointed out that matrix vesicles are only found associated with the initial calcification of cartilage, woven bone and first-formed dentine. Questions arise as to the continued mineralization of these tissues and to the onset of mineralization in mineralized tissue, such as cement and enamel where matrix vesicles cannot be demonstrated. One suggestion is that as these latter two tissues form on previously mineralized tissue (dentine): crystal initiation spreads from crystals in the dentine. A suggestion with more support is that in bone and dentine (and probably cement) the non-collagenous constituents of the organic matrix have a role to play. Two such constituents have been implicated, a protein called *osteonectin* which has the ability to bind to both collagen and hydroxyapatite and a *phosphoprotein* which some workers believe binds to calcium. Even so, conclusive proof that these proteins represent heterogeneous nucleation sites has not been forthcoming. Then there are

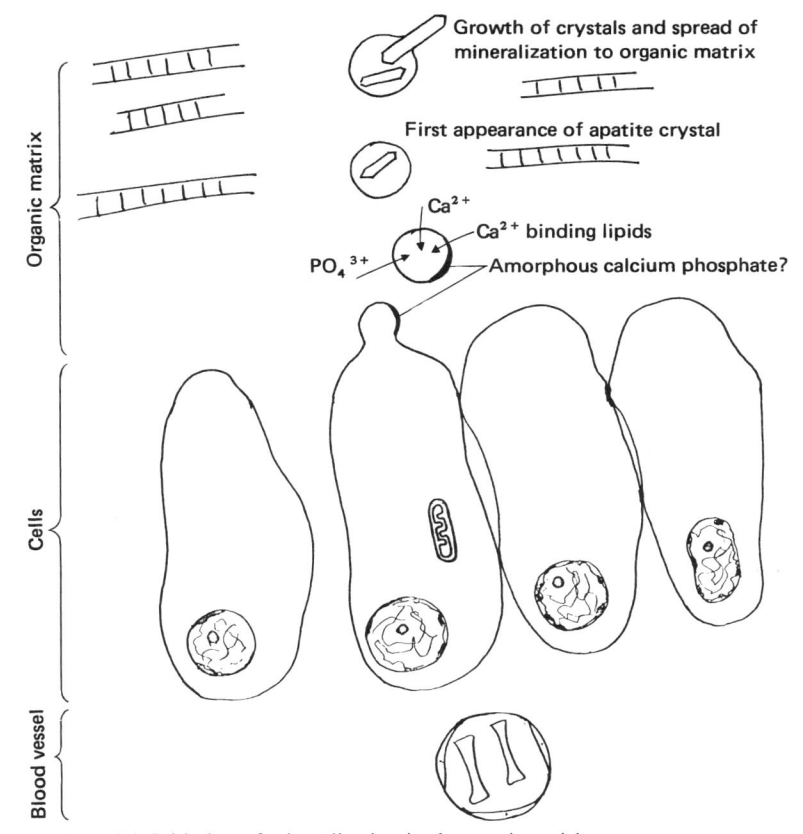

Fig. 10.3. Initiation of mineralization in the matrix vesicle.

published electron micrographs showing the first apatite crystals appearing in a periodic fashion coincident with the periodicity of collagen (*Fig. 10.4*). Whether such a picture indicates the presence of a nucleation site on the collagen molecule or the site where a protein such as osteonectin binds with collagen has not been determined. Once initial crystals have been formed by heterogeneous nucleation, the number of crystals can increase by secondary nucleation which is the formation of additional crystals nucleated by the mineral phase particles already formed, or by further heterogeneous nucleation. Accepting the initial appearance of apatite in matrix vesicles and in association with the collagen fibrils, there is no doubt that subsequently the majority of the mineral in bone and dentine is developed by crystal growth.

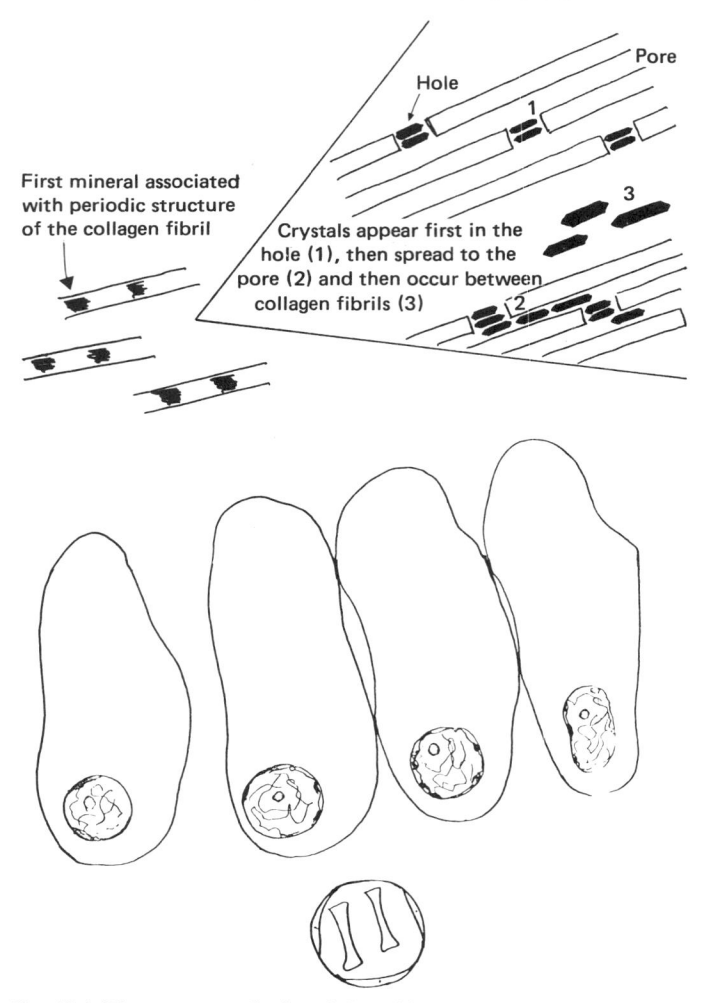

Fig. 10.4. The sequence of mineral deposition associated with the collagen fibril.

Alkaline Phosphatase

Crystal growth is inhibited by the accumulation of pyrophosphate on its surface and this must be removed if growth is to continue. The enzyme *alkaline phosphatase* is thought to achieve this. Alkaline phosphatase is the name given to a group of hydrolytic enzymes, described as orthophosphoric monoester phosphohydrolysases, which function by liberating inorganic phosphate from phosphate esters. They have been believed to be associated with the process of mineralization for nearly 60 years when it was first postulated that the enzyme at mineralizing sites released inorganic phosphate from ester phosphates and that the local elevation of phosphate ions resulted in the precipitation of bone mineral. However, to this day the exact role of the enzyme in mineralization has not been properly determined. In addition to the role of pyrophosphate removal already mentioned, it is suggested that the enzyme is associated with the transfer of phosphate ions (and also calcium ions) across cell membranes. It has already been pointed out that the enzymes can often be demonstrated where ions are transferred across a membrane and it is known that the enzyme itself can become phosphorylated at low pHs; this could lead to the formation of specific sites for transporting phosphates. *Figure 10.5* shows the location of this enzyme in mineralizing regions and indicates the possible function at each location.

Crystallite Localization

Another problem related to mineralization is the location of the apatite crystal in the organic matrix. It is known, for example, that 70–80 per cent of the mineral in bone exists within the collagen fibrils. Chapter 9 explained that gaps or holes are present in the collagen fibril as well as pores which are the spaces between adjacent molecules. During mineralization the crystals first appear in the holes, only later in the pores, and finally in the extracellular compartment between the fibrils (*Fig. 10.4*). What is not known is whether the mineralization is due entirely to heterogeneous nucleation or secondary nucleation from the crystals deposited in the holes.

COMPARISONS

Having outlined in fairly simple terms the salient features of hard tissue genesis (summarized in *Fig. 10.6*) it is a rewarding exercise to examine the formation of the individual hard tissues to see how closely they are comparable. At the same time such a comparison should emphasize the similar principles involved in the genesis of each tissue.

Bones can be formed by either intramembranous or endochondral ossification. But the actual formation of bone tissue is fundamentally the same because, although in endochondral formation the bone is preceded by a cartilaginous model, this is replaced by bone deposited in the same way as in the intramembranous situation. Bone is mineralized connective tissue and its formation (intramembranous bone formation) is heralded by an increase in local vascularity of the mesenchyme. At the same time the cells of the mesenchyme in this area differentiate into distinctive cells called osteoblasts. These cells are rich in RNA associated with a well-developed rough endoplasmic reticulum and have a well-developed

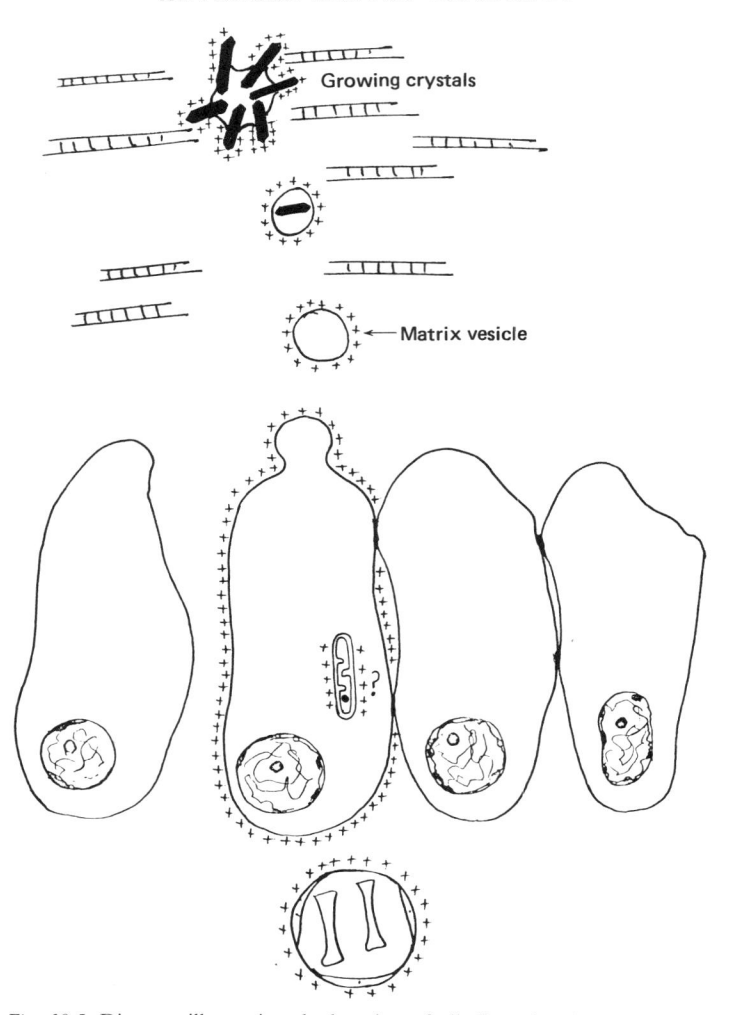

Fig. 10.5. Diagram illustrating the location of alkaline phosphatase activity (+ + +) in the formation of a mineralized tissue.

Golgi apparatus and alkaline phosphatase activity. They synthesize the ground substance and the forerunners of the collagen molecule (procollagen) which is assembled extracellularly into collagen fibrils in the ground substance. The collagen fibrils and the ground substance constitute the organic matrix of unmineralized bone (osteoid), and it is into this that mineral salts are deposited. The first foci of mineral salts in the organic matrix are related to matrix vesicles formed from protoplasmic buds of

HARD TISSUE GENESIS

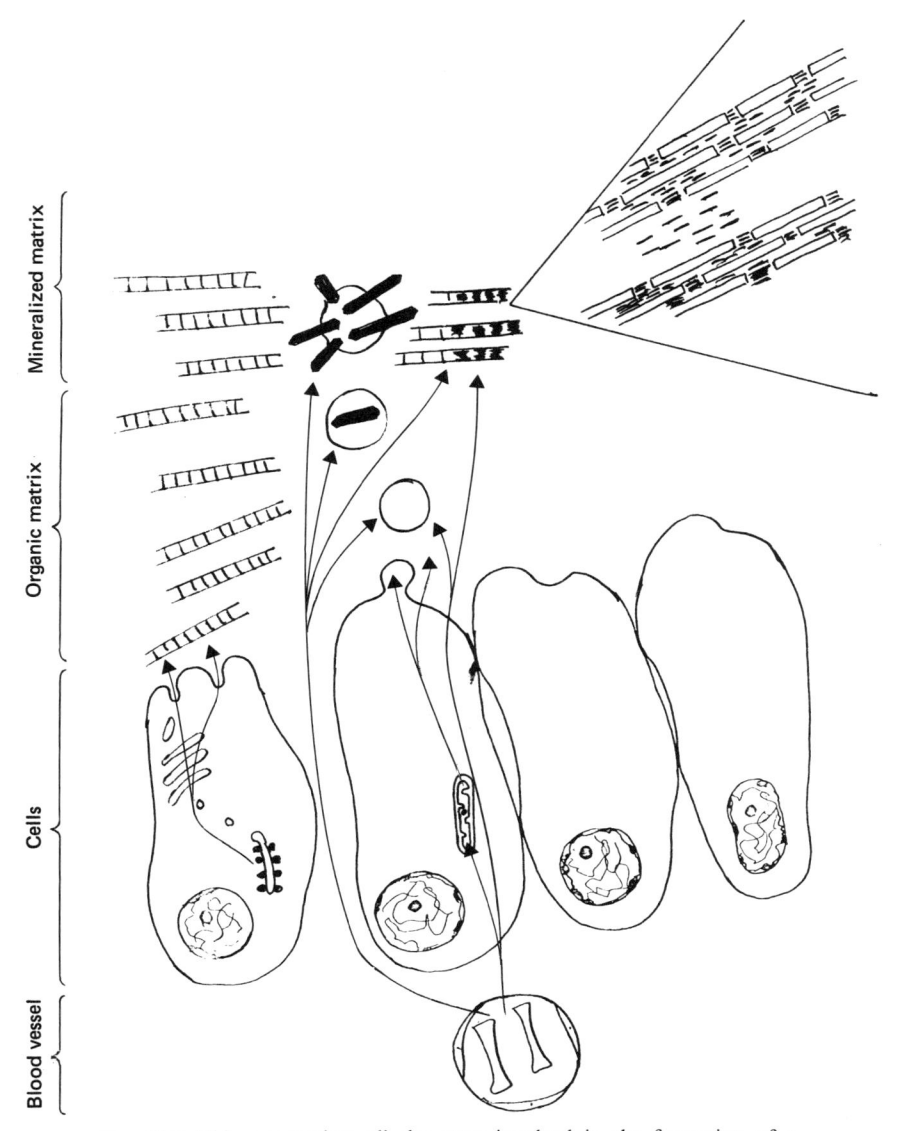

Fig. 10.6. This summarizes all the steps involved in the formation of a mineralized tissue and is a combination of *Figs. 10.1–10.5.*

the osteoblasts. Continued crystal growth from these foci results in the osteoblast becoming surrounded by mineralized matrix and the cell is then termed an 'osteocyte'. *Figure 10.7* illustrates this sequence of events and it

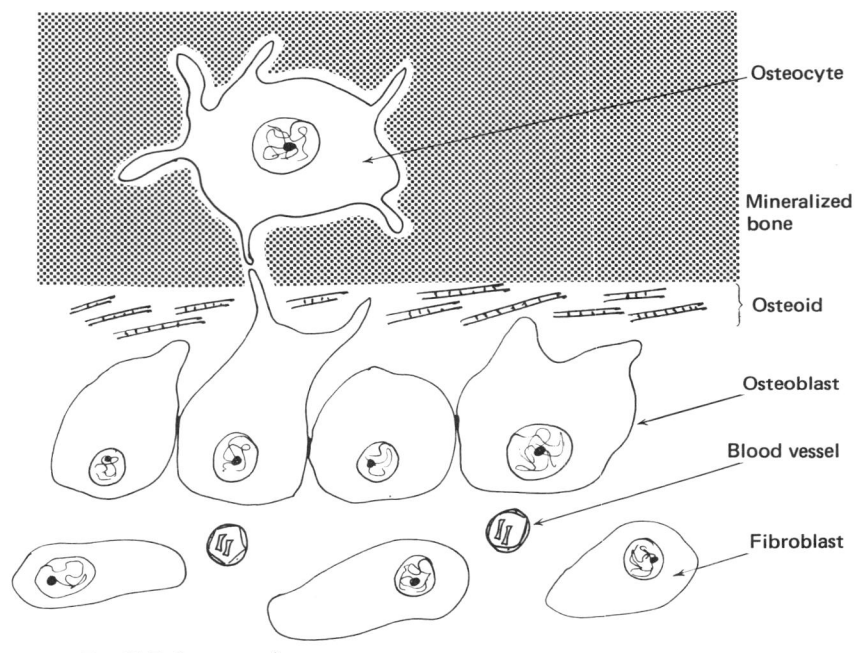

Fig. 10.7. Osteogenesis.

will be seen that it is essentially similar to *Fig. 10.1*, differing only in that the bone-forming cells become trapped within the forming hard tissue. In endochondral bone formation the cartilage model is invaded by vascular mesenchymal osteogenic tissue which elaborates bone in essentially the same way. However, there is one significant difference; when the cartilage model is invaded by osteogenic tissue the cartilage mineralizes and provides the scaffold for the forming bone. In this situation the newly formed osteoid does not seem to mineralize by the provision of matrix vesicles. Instead, the tissue mineralizes by crystal growth from the pre-existing crystallites in the mineralized cartilage. It must be pointed out that this account of bone formation applies to the coarse-fibred embryonic bone which later undergoes remodelling to be replaced by adult fine-fibred bone.

The formation of cement is almost identical to that of bone. Cement is also a mineralized connective tissue and is formed by cementoblasts, the cement-forming cells, which differentiate from the ectomesenchymal dental follicle surrounding the developing root. These cells are almost identical to osteoblasts and they elaborate the collagen fibrils and ground substance of the unmineralized cement matrix (precement = cementoid). The cementoblasts may or may not be incorporated in the mineralizing matrix and this determines the two types of cement seen in histological sections, acellular and cellular. *Figure 10.8* gives the essential details of cementogenesis. As cement is always laid down over the pre-existing dentine, it is thought that the initial mineralization of the cementoid takes place by crystal growth from the mineralized dentine.

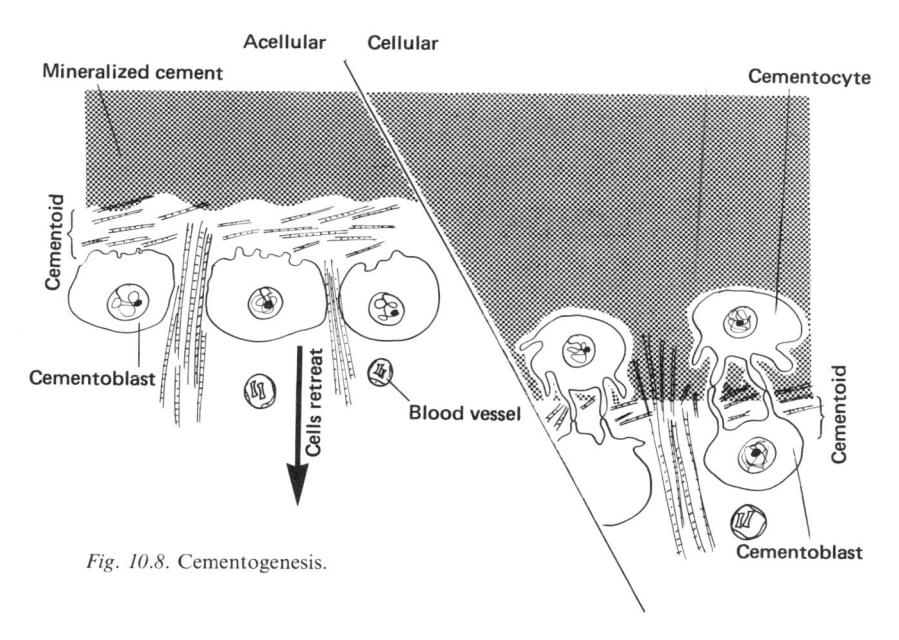

Fig. 10.8. Cementogenesis.

Like cement, dentine is also formed from ectomesenchymal connective tissue but it differs significantly from bone and cement, especially in its structural features. Even so, the principles underlying its formation are the same. Specialized cells, the odontoblasts, differentiate from the cells of the dental papilla after induction by the cells of the internal dental epithelium. At the same time other papillary cells congregate beneath the newly differentiated odontoblasts, forming the sub-odontoblast layer in which exists a capillary plexus from which capillary loops pass into the odontoblast layer. The newly differentiated odontoblasts develop an extensive endoplasmic reticulum, a prominent Golgi apparatus and exhibit marked oxidative and alkaline phosphatase activity around the plasma membrane. This enzyme is also found in the cells of the sub-odontoblast layer. The odontoblasts form the organic matrix of dentine and at the same time retreat towards the centre of the papilla, each leaving behind a slender process which becomes surrounded by matrix. The dentine matrix becomes mineralized to form tubular dentine (*Fig. 10.9*). The odontoblasts in this situation, like the osteoblasts in membranous ossification, have cellular buds which become matrix vesicles and provide the foci for mineralization.

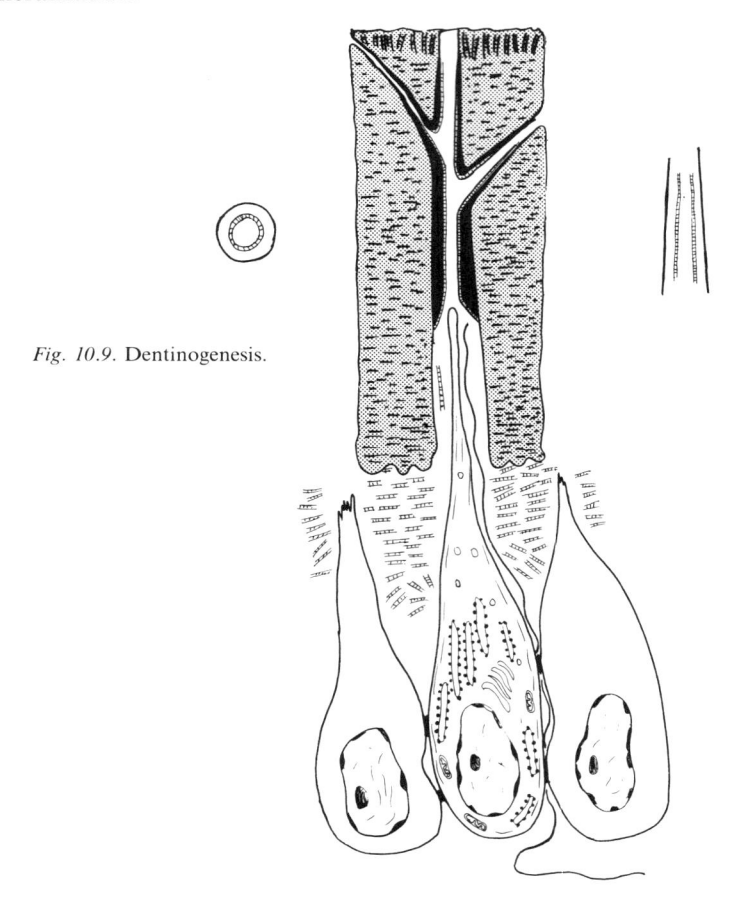

Fig. 10.9. Dentinogenesis.

Thus far, therefore, it is evident that osteogenesis, cementogenesis and dentinogenesis have many common features. These hard tissues are all specialized forms of connective tissue; they all develop in areas of high vascularity; specialized cells are associated with the formation of the organic matrix which consists of collagen fibrils and a ground substance. The cells have common ultrastructural and enzymatic features and mineralization occurs within the organic matrix.

When amelogenesis is considered, it would appear that enamel formation differs significantly from that of the other hard tissues. Enamel is an epidermal product and for this reason its organic matrix does not contain collagen. By analogy with the fibrous collagen scaffolding of other mesenchymal hard tissues it was once assumed that enamel employed a fibrous protein, keratin, to fulfil the same function. However, this is now known not to be the case and, although no fibrous component is involved in enamel matrix formation, amelogenesis can be shown to be closely similar in principle to the formation of other hard tissues.

The histology of amelogenesis, outlined in *Fig. 10.10*, shows that two cellular elements are involved, the enamel-forming cells or ameloblasts and the cells of the stratum intermedium. The latter are exceptionally rich in alkaline phosphatase activity and the ameloblasts are rich in RNA and have a high activity of oxidative enzymes. If the ultrastructure of the ameloblast is examined, its features are essentially similar to those of the osteoblast or odontoblast in that there is a well-developed rough endoplasmic reticulum, Golgi apparatus, many mitochondria and secretory vesicles. In other words, it has the characteristics of a protein-synthesizing and -secreting cell.

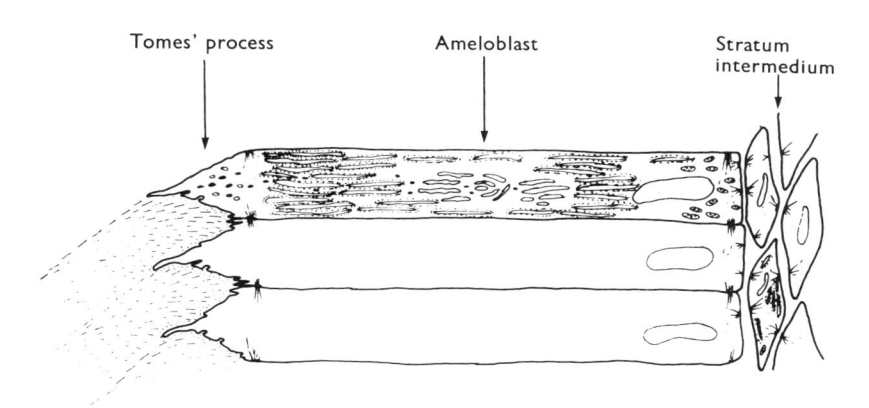

Fig. 10.10. Amelogenesis.

In view of the once-supposed presence of keratinous material in enamel matrix, it is interesting to compare the ultrastructure of the ameloblast with that of the keratin-producing cell. The keratinizing cell has very little rough endoplasmic reticulum but instead has many free ribosomes. The protein synthesized in this cell is retained and aggregated in a fibrous form, so that the cytoplasm eventually becomes laden with keratin. Such a cell is described as a protein-synthesizing and -retaining cell and it is clear that the ameloblast does not fall into this category. Thus far amelogenesis corresponds to the genesis of the other hard tissues. Blood vessels are present, adjacent to the outer dental epithelium, the enzymatic picture corresponds and the formative cell secretes a proteinaceous material which forms the organic matrix. However, when discussing amelogenesis later in this book, evidence will be presented showing that this organic matrix does not become organized into a fibrous form but remains in the form of a gel. Into this organic mineral salts are deposited almost coincident with the secretion of matrix. There is no evidence for any matrix vesicles associated with the ameloblast.

It is apparent, then, that the hard tissues, irrespective of their derivation, reveal similar principles in their genesis. These may be summarized as the production of an organic matrix by cells which exhibit protein synthesizing and secreting features, and introduction into this matrix of mineral salts. It is suggested that where mineralization is occurring for the first time, such as in membranous bone formation, dentine formation and in mineralizing cartilage, the foci for initial appearance of inorganic crystals are vesicles which bud from the cell and provide a local environment for initiation. Where hard tissue genesis is taking place in association with pre-existing mineralized tissue, for example, cement in relation to mineralized dentine, bone in relation to mineralized cartilage and enamel in relation to mineralized dentine, mineralization occurs in the newly formed matrix by crystal growth from the pre-existing mineralized tissue.

REFERENCES AND FURTHER READING

References pertinent to this chapter can be found following the chapters on Dentinogenesis (Chapter 12), Amelogenesis (Chapter 15) and Cementogenesis and Cement Structure (Chapter 17).

An up-to-date review can be found in Veis A. (ed.) (1982), 'The Chemistry and Biology of Mineralized Tissues', *Development in Biochemistry*, vol. 22. New York, Elsevier-North Holland Inc.

CHAPTER 11

BONE

This chapter does not attempt to deal with the detailed histology of bone for which the reader is referred to any standard histology textbook. Rather we present one or two aspects of bone not normally considered in such sources but which are of some significance in clarifying terminology and explaining such phenomena as tooth movement and facial growth.

When bone tissue is first formed, or when it is rapidly laid down, for example in the embryo and in the repair of wounds, the preexisting connective tissue of the area is colonized by new bone. The collagen in the connective tissue and the collagen elaborated by the newly differentiated bone-forming cells, the osteoblasts, together form the fibrous matrix of this new bone. As a result the collagen fibres are of varying thickness and orientation and many are continuous with the collagen fibres of the adjacent soft connective tissue. This type of bone is termed 'coarse-fibred woven bone' or 'embryonic bone' and is laid down in trabeculae or plates which surround areas of soft connective tissue (*Fig. 11.1*).

From this starting point woven bone is remodelled to form mature bone. In mature bone the collagen fibres of the matrix are of even thickness and are laid down in sheets or lamellae. In each lamella the collagen fibres are all orientated in one direction, although the orientation and number of collagen fibres vary from lamella to lamella. Lamellae of

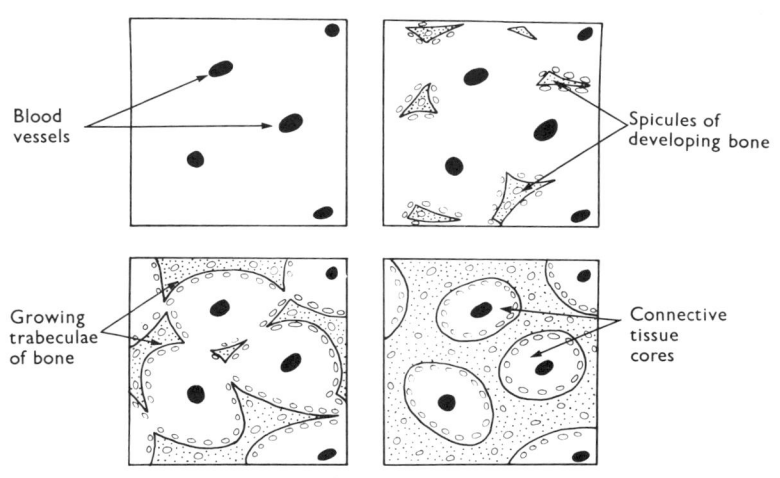

Fig. 11.1. Four stages in the formation of embryonic (woven, immature, coarse-fibred) bone.

bone are laid down in two ways. They can be laid down concentrically (from outside to inside) to form osteons (Haversian systems) or in sheets on the surface of bones as circumferential lamellae. Embryonic bone is replaced by mature bone as follows. Between the trabeculae of woven bone is soft connective tissue with its associated blood vessels. On the internal surface of the trabeculae new bone is laid down in layers or lamellae with the result that, as each layer is laid down, the volume of the unmineralized connective tissue is diminished until only a small core, which transmits blood vessels, remains. This osteon formed within woven bone is termed a 'primary' osteon (*Fig. 11.2*). The primary osteon has a periphery which is ill defined when viewed in the light microscope because the collagen fibres here are continuous with those of the woven bone. Also the cells in the primary osteon are larger and have a somewhat irregular disposition. Thus we now have a form of bone which consists of a mixture of woven bone, primary osteons and circumferential bone at its periphery.

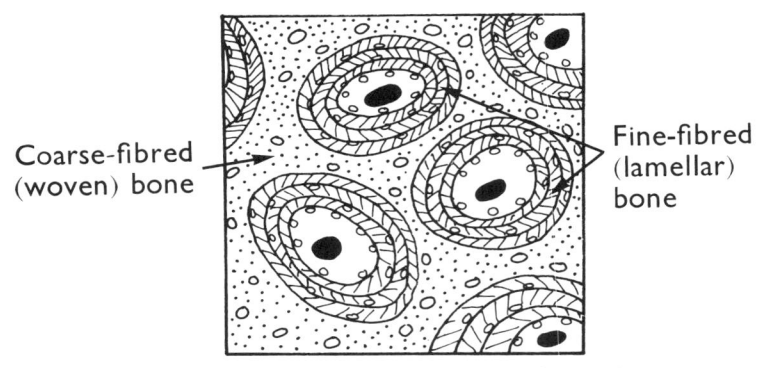

Fig. 11.2. Primary osteons form within the trabeculae of woven bone.

From this point on, either mature compact (adult) bone or mature cancellous (adult) bone is developed. These two types of bone can be distinguished by their ratios of hard and soft connective tissue. Thus compact bone consists of comparatively solid blocks of bone in which the proportion of mineralized tissue is far greater than the proportion of soft connective tissue, whereas in cancellous bone the blocks of bone are separated by a considerable portion of soft connective tissue and macroscopically have a honeycomb appearance. Mature bone is formed by a process of careful remodelling where resorption first takes place indiscriminately within the trabeculae of primary osteons and woven bone. The area resorbed is replaced by soft connective tissue. Within the concavity of the resorbed area bone is laid down, in a similar manner as described for the primary osteon, to form what is termed the 'secondary osteon' (*Fig. 11.3*). The secondary osteon is marked at its periphery by a reversal line which indicates the extent of resorption. Depending on the amount of remodelling and infilling of the soft connective tissue spaces, either mature cancellous or mature compact bone is formed. During remodelling, remnants of previous osteons remain and these are termed 'interstitial bone'.

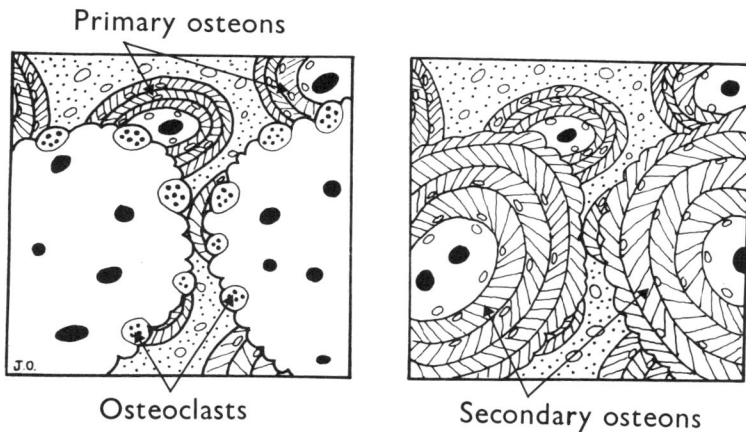

Fig. 11.3. The conversion of embryonic bone into adult bone; the formation of secondary osteons.

It must be realized that the above account is somewhat simplified and transitional forms of bone are often seen. In summary, however, we can consider compact bone as consisting of surface or circumferential lamellar bone, primary and secondary (tertiary and so on) osteons and interstitial bone—the latter consisting of either remnants of previous osteons or of parts of other osteons. The relative amounts of each vary considerably in samples of compact bone from different sources. Cancellous or trabecular bone has a similar structure to compact bone but differs in that complete osteons are fewer and there is a much greater amount of interstitial bone.

This account of bone development should make an understanding of bone terminology a little easier. This terminology is somewhat confusing because of the several different ways of classifying bone. *Figure 11.4* summarizes the ways in which bone has been classified. The figure explains why fine-fibred lamellar bone is found in Haversian system bone and in compact bone; why Haversian system bone is found in cancellous bone. A simple way to remember the differing classifications of bone is to relate each classification to an order of magnification, namely with the naked eye, with a low-power lens and with a high-power lens.

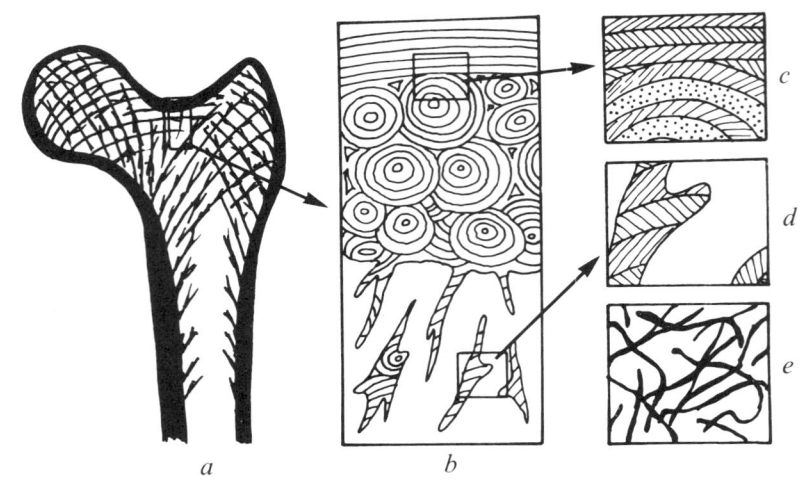

Fig. 11.4. Some terms used in the description of bone tissue. *a*, Viewed with the naked eye bone appears to be either compact or cancellous (=spongy or trabecular). The compact layer forms the cortex of the bone; hence the term 'cortical bone'. *b*, Viewed with a low-power lens the deeper region of the compact (=cortical) bone is seen to consist of Haversian systems (=osteons) in which layers (=lamellae) of bone are arranged concentrically around each central canal of the system. At the periphery of the compact layer, the lamellae are arranged circumferentially around the surface of the whole bone. Therefore compact bone contains concentric, circumferential and, in the spaces, interstitial lamellae. It will be noted that the trabeculae in spongy bone are also composed of lamellae. All (nearly) the bone in an adult is built up of lamellae (*c, d*) in which the collagen fibres are regular and fine. In adjacent lamellae the fibres run in different directions (some fibres are often cut transversely, appearing as dots in a section: *c*). Therefore, adult bone is both fine-fibred and lamellated. In contrast, woven (=embryonic) bone contains coarse, irregularly arranged fibres (*e*).

From the above account it is evident, therefore, that a considerable amount of internal remodelling by means of resorption and deposition occurs within bone.

The remodelling of surface bone plays a significant part in bone growth. Surface remodelling is brought about in the same way as internal remodelling, namely by means of controlled sites of bone deposition and bone resorption utilizing the same cellular bases, the osteoblast and the osteoclast.

An appreciation of both the nature and extent of bone remodelling explains its remarkable plasticity seen during development. The constant deposition and removal of bone tissue, again and again, accommodates the growth of a bone without changing its shape, function or relation to neighbouring structures. Thus, for example, a significant increase in size of the mandible is achieved from birth to maturity largely by bony remodelling without any loss in function or change in its relative position in the maxilla. It is most unlikely that any of the bone tissue present in the 1-year-old mandible is present in the same bone 30 years later.

REFERENCES AND FURTHER READING

For further reading on the structure and function of bone the three volumes of *The Biochemistry and Physiology of Bone,* edited by G. H. Bourne (New York, Academic, 1972) and *The Physiology of Bone* 3rd ed. by J. M. Vaughan (Oxford, Clarendon Press, 1981 are recommended.

CHAPTER 12

DENTINOGENESIS

The formation of dentine begins at the late bell stage of tooth development and is a function of the dental papilla. Cells become differentiated at the periphery of the papilla and they form and mineralize an organic matrix which becomes dentine. These cells are called odontoblasts.

Before differentiation of odontoblasts occurs the short columnar cells of the internal dental epithelium become tall columnar and their nuclei move to the ends of the cells away from the papilla. These changes have been equated with the differentiation of dentine-forming cells in the papilla as tissue culture studies have shown unequivocally that the differentiation of these cells is induced by epithelium. However, in terms of induction, the significance of these morphological changes in the internal dental epithelium have been over-emphasized for a similar induction of papilla cells takes place during root formation without any changes occurring in the epithelial cells. The histological changes which occur in the enamel epithelium are in fact preparatory to the cells assuming their function of enamel formation.

The newly differentiated odontoblast is characterized histologically by its location and its size; histochemically by its high RNA content and marked oxidative and hydrolytic enzyme activity and ultrastructurally by a well-developed Golgi complex, numerous mitochondria, many vesicular structures and a well-developed microtubular system. As the odontoblasts differentiate there is also an increase in the number of papillal cells immediately subjacent and these form the sub-odontoblast layer, a feature of which is a high level of alkaline phosphatase activity. This enzyme is also associated with the plasma membranes of the odontoblasts. When odontoblasts first differentiate they are surrounded by an extensive extracellular compartment consisting of ground substance containing very few, if any, fine collagen fibres which, as the odontoblasts continue to hypertrophy, is gradually diminished until finally cell-to-cell contacts are established between adjacent odontoblasts. In that portion of the extracellular compartment adjacent to the basement membranes supporting the internal dental epithelium large-diameter collagen fibrils appear generally arranged at right angles to the basement membrane. These fibres are formed by the odontoblasts and, together with the ground substance, constitute the initial dentine matrix. At the same time the odontoblast begins to move away towards the centre of the dental papilla and from its trailing edge a number of matrix vesicles and short stubby processes are pushed out towards the basement membrane associated with the internal dental epithelium. One of these processes persists as the odontoblast

DENTINOGENESIS

continues to migrate and forms a principal extension, the odontoblast process, which eventually comes to occupy a tubule in the formed dentine. Thus, the first few microns or so of dentine matrix deposited against the basal laminae of the internal dental epithelium consist of a milieu of ground substance containing large-diameter collagen fibres aligned perpendicular to the basement membrane, protoplasmic extensions of the odontoblast and matrix vesicles. The pattern of collagen fibril deposition soon changes so that much finer diameter collagen fibrils are now deposited, along with ground substance, and are arranged in a plane parallel to the basement membranes. This arrangement continues as the rest of, and therefore the bulk of, the dentine is formed. This means that, on the basis of collagen fibre orientation and size, two types of dentine can be recognized: mantle dentine which is the first-formed dentine adjacent to the internal dental epithelium and the remainder of the dentine called circumpulpal dentine (*Fig. 12.1*). There is a distinction between coronal mantle dentine and root mantle dentine which has only been appreciated recently and relates to the orientation of the coarse collagen fibres. In root mantle dentine these fibres are aligned parallel with, instead of perpendicular to, the basal lamina supporting the epithelium which in the root is Hertwig's epithelial root sheath (*Fig. 12.2*).

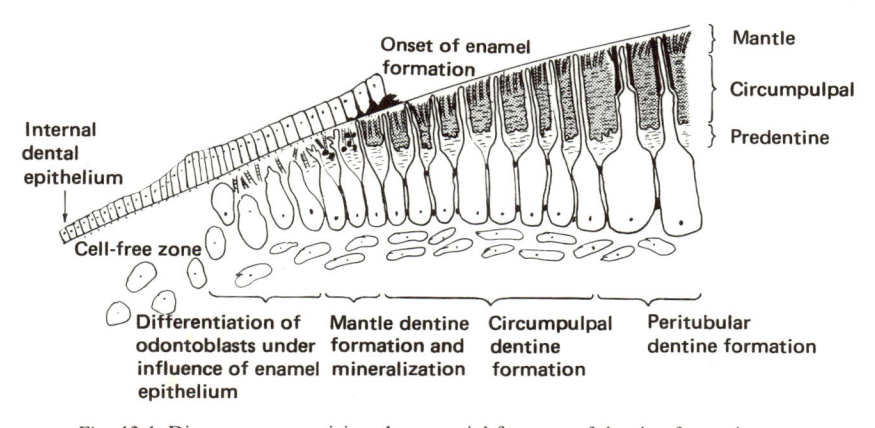

Fig. 12.1. Diagram summarizing the essential features of dentine formation.

The formation of dentine collagen has been well studied because the polarized nature of the odontoblast makes it a useful model system and a great deal of basic information relating to collagen synthesis has come from such study. Using techniques such as autoradiography and immunohistochemistry in association with the electron microscope, the route for

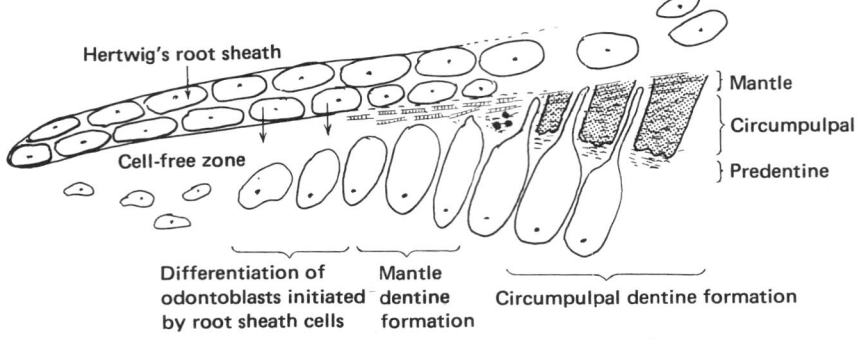

Fig. 12.2. Diagram illustrating root dentinogenesis which is similar to coronal dentinogenesis except for the large-diameter collagen fibrils in mantle dentine.

collagen synthesis via the ribosomes of the RER, the Golgi complex, secretory vesicles and thence to the cell surface (*see* Chapter 10) was established as also was the transit time of about 35 minutes.

The Problem of von Korff Fibres

From the account given here it is evident that all the collagen of the dentine matrix forms as a result of odontoblast activity. This is a recent appreciation as previously it was thought that there was a dual origin for dentine matrix collagen with mantle dentine collagen forming from the activity of the cells of the sub-odontoblast layer and circumpulpal dentine collagen forming as a result of odontoblast activity. The cells of the sub-odontoblast layer were thought to form large collagen fibre bundles which passed between the odontoblasts in a spiral fashion as the fibres of von Korff which then fanned out against the surface of the basal lamina of the internal dental epithelium to form the fibrillar component of mantle dentine (*Fig. 12.3*). Some believe (and it is the view expressed here) that von Korff fibres are an artefact of the light microscope. When thick sections of a developing tooth (50 µm) are stained with silver and examined with the light microscope the classic picture of many argyrophilic (silver-loving) von Korff fibres related to initial dentinogenesis are seen decreasing in number during dentinogenesis. If this same thick section is now sectioned again and examined with the electron microscope, von Korff fibres cannot be identified. Only small particles of silver in an extensive extracellular compartment are seen. If similar sections are pretreated with acetic anhydride, which blocks reducing sugars, this silver staining is also abolished. This indicates that the silver is captured by the reducing sugars of the ground substances. How then can these observations be correlated with the presence of von Korff fibres? Presumably

DENTINOGENESIS

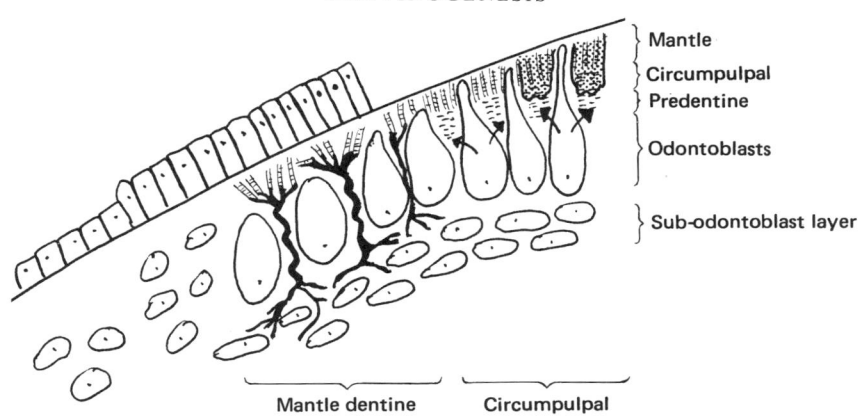

Fig. 12.3. Diagram illustrating the supposed dual origin of dentine matrix collagen. Mantle dentine collagen is thought to come from activity of the cells of the subodontoblast layer whereas circumpulpal dentine collagen is the result of odontoblastic activity.

the extensive intercellular compartment between the newly differentiated odontoblasts contains reducing sugars which become impregnated with silver. When viewed with the light microscope, a negative outline of the odontoblasts results and this gives a simulated appearance of fibres (*Fig. 12.4*). This explanation of the so-called von Korff fibres also explains their diminution when circupulpal dentinogenesis begins. As the odontoblasts hypertrophy, they become more closely packed together, develop junctions and eliminate most of the extracellular compartment between them. Hence there can be no extracellular deposition of silver and no von Korff fibres.

The large-diameter fibres found in mantle dentine are often referred to as von Korff fibres and, if this term is to be retained, it should be emphasized that it refers to fibres confined to the mantle dentine and which originate from odontoblastic activity.

A question which is still unresolved is why large-diameter fibres are restricted to mantle dentine and an explanation may be that first-formed collagen of dentine is aggregated within an extracellular compartment abundant in ground substance, whereas in later dentinogenesis the collagen is aggregated in an environment with minimal ground substance.

Mineralization

Thus, the role of the odontoblast in the formation of the organic matrix of dentine is fairly well understood. The manner whereby mineral salts are introduced into this matrix is now also better understood. The organic matrix is always formed first so that there is always a layer of predentine

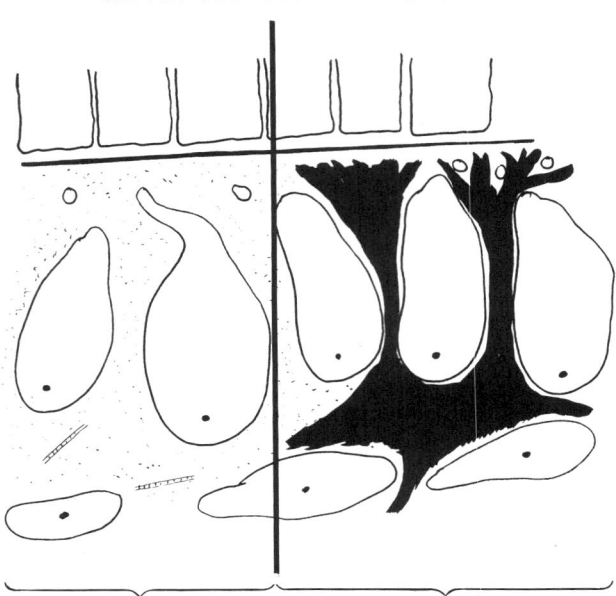

Early dentinogenesis as seen with the electron microscope The odontoblasts are separated by an extracellular compartment which is ground-substance rich and collagen fibril poor. When stained with silver the reducing sugars of the ground substance capture the silver (black dots)

In a thick section the silver salts in the extracellular compartment amass to form a dense mass which mimic fibres between the cells. This silver staining is abolished if sections are first treated to block the reducing sugars

Fig. 12.4. Diagram illustrating the artefactural nature of the von Korff fibres.

(unmineralized matrix) adjacent to the odontoblasts. In mantle dentine matrix vesicles have been clearly identified functioning in the manner described in Chapter 10 and providing the initial focus of mineralization for dentine. Matrix vesicles are not found during circumpulpal dentinogenesis and continued mineralization of the organic matrix must therefore be either by crystal growth or by heterogeneous nucleation. In dentine phospholipids and phosphoproteins have been implicated as possible nucleators as also has the collagen molecule.

The route taken by calcium ions to the mineralizing front is also debatable although recent studies using pyroantimonate as a marker for calcium suggest that an intracellular route is the preferred pathway; alkaline phosphatase activity has been demonstrated associated with the cell membrane of the odontoblasts and its activity has been linked to calcium transfer into the cell. An accumulation of mitrochondrial calcium granules prior to the onset of dentine mineralization also occurs.

Peritubular Dentine

Examination of the fine structure of dentine reveals the presence of a sheath of more highly mineralized peritubular dentine around the odontoblast process (*Fig. 12.5*). The first appearance of the peritubular dentine is in the fully mineralized dentine matrix near the predentine-dentine border and coincides with the narrowing in width of the odontoblast process; the peritubular dentine thus occupies some of the space formerly occupied by the odontoblast process. Little is known about the genesis of the peritubular dentine. However, there are certain features of the odontoblast, its processes and the peritubular dentine which permit some speculation.

There are morphological features of the odontoblast and its process which can be equated, in part, with synthesis of the peritubular dentine.

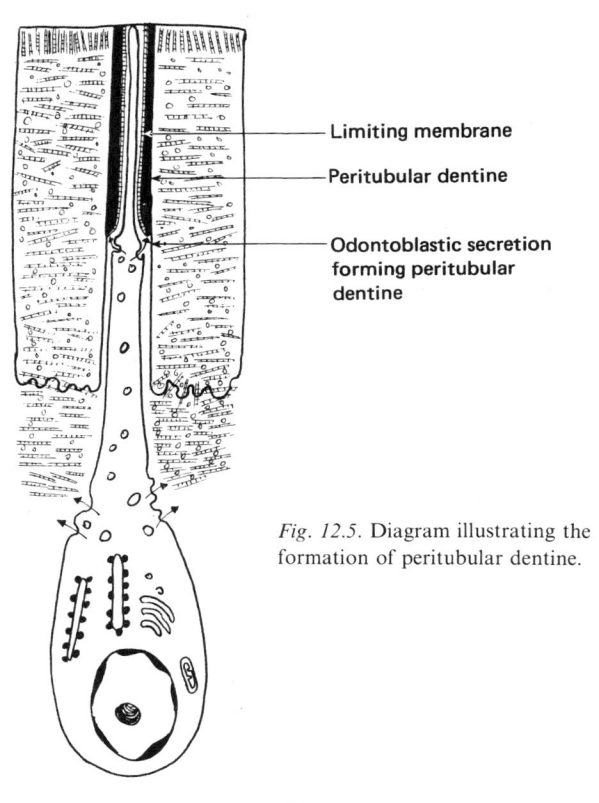

Fig. 12.5. Diagram illustrating the formation of peritubular dentine.

Thus, the odontoblasts process contains a well-developed system of microtubules, vesicular structures and surface bays, which have, in other situations, been equated with transport and secretory mechanisms. The presence of such structures within the odontoblast process explains how peritubular dentine formation occurs within the depths of already-formed dentine. Material synthesized by the odontoblast cell body passes via the process to the site of the peritubular dentine formation. However, the above features might merely demonstrate activity of odontoblasts unrelated to the development of peritubular dentine. In this case, peritubular dentine formation would involve a redistribution of dentine mineral in response to purely physiochemical changes. This view is supported by an unpublished observation (Osborn) that the hardness of translucent dentine is the same as that of adjacent 'normal' dentine.

Tubule Shape

Another interesting aspect of dentinogenesis is the course taken by the odontoblasts as they retreat towards the centre of the pulp. As they leave behind them a process which is incorporated in the mineralized matrix, examination of the tubules of mature dentine provides a permanent record of the path taken by the individual odontoblasts. It is known that the tubules have a primary S-shaped curvature and also secondary curvatures.

There is a hypothesis to explain the genesis of these curvatures. It has been suggested that the primary curvatures result from the oscillations of the odontoblasts which arise from their crowding as the volume of the pulp decreases. This has been tested by a simple model experiment. The outline of the dentine surface of a tooth in longitudinal section is traced on smoked paper. If beads, representing the odontoblasts, are aligned along the periphery of the drawing and progressively pushed in a centripetal direction, starting with those beneath the cusp tip, the sinuous tracks so produced on the smoked paper mimic the primary curvatures of the dentinal tubules (*Fig. 12.6*). At the same time, it will be seen that the beads become progressively more crowded as they move centripetally. The origin of the secondary curvatures is more difficult to explain, but a tentative solution has been offered. This is based upon the accepted observations that enamel spindles are most frequently encountered beneath the tips of cusps, where crowding of the retreating odontoblasts is most intense. Under such conditions, it is suggested that in unit time the formed length of the odontoblast process is greater than the distance moved by the odontoblast towards the papilla (*Fig. 12.7*). Hence, the process might become buckled and the secondary curvatures established. In marsupials the odontoblasts send processes through the full thickness of the enamel (producing enamel tubules). This indicates that odontoblasts can produce a greater length of process than the distance they move.

DENTINOGENESIS

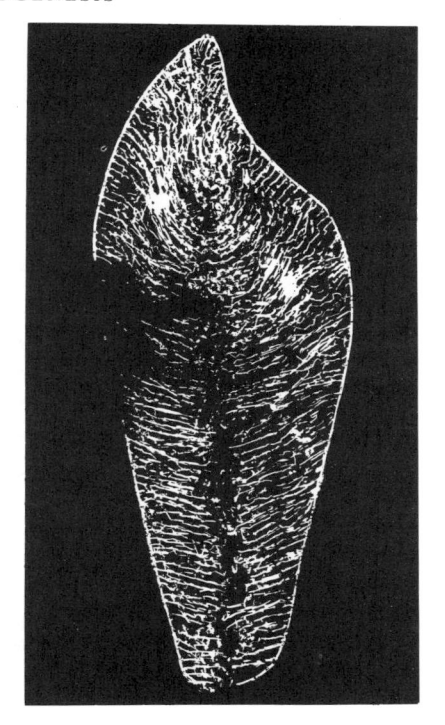

Fig. 12.6. Scratch marks made on smoked card by beads simulating the primary curvatures of dentine tubules.

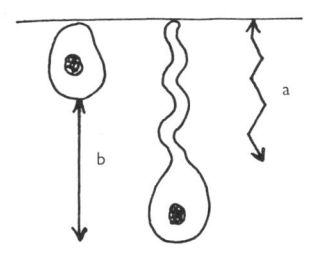

Fig. 12.7. Distance, *a*, the true length of the forming odontoblast process, is greater than *b*, the distance moved by the odontoblast in the same time.

REFERENCES AND FURTHER READING

Bevelander G. (1941) The development and structure of the fiber system of dentine. *Anat. Rec.* **81**, 79.

Bevelander G. and Hiroshi N. (1966) The formation and mineralization of dentine. *Anat. Rec.* **156**, 303.

von Ebner V. (1906) Ueber die Entwicklung der leimgebenden Fibrillen im Zahnbein (Development of collagenous fibrils in the dentine). *Sitzungsber. Akad. Wissensch. Vienna*, **115**, 281; *Anat. Anz.* **29**, 137.

Eisenmann D. R. and Glick P. L. (1972) Ultrastructure of initial crystal formation in dentine. *J. Ultrastruct. Res.* **41**, 18.

Garant P. R., Zabo G. and Nalbandian J. (1968) The fine structure of the mouse odontoblast. *Arch. Oral Biol.* **13**, 857.

Harrop T. J. and Mackay B. (1968) Electron microscopic observations on healing in the dental pulp in the rat. *Arch. Oral Biol.* **13**, 365.

Herold R. C. and Kaye H. (1966) Mitochondria in odontoblastic processes. *Nature, Lond.* **210**, 108.

von Korff K. (1905) Die Entwicklung der Zahnbein und Knockengrundsubstanz der Sangetiere. *Arch. Mikrosk. Anat. EntwMech.* **67**, 1.

Kramer, I. R. H. (1951) The distribution of collagen fibrils in the dentine matrix. *Br. Dent. J.* **91**, 1.

Lenz H. (1969) Elektonenmikroskopische Untersuchungen der Dentinentwicklung (Electron microscopic studies of dentine development). *Dtsch. Zahn. Mund. Kieferheilk.* **30**, 367.

Lester K. S. (1969) The unusual nature of root formation in molar teeth of the laboratory rat. *J. Ultrastruct. Res.* **28**, 481.

Lester K. S. and Boyde A. (1968) The question of von Korff fibres in mammalian dentine. *Calc. Tiss. Res.* **1**, 273.

Moss M. L. (1974) Studies on dentine. I. Mantle dentine. *Acta Anat.* **87**, 481.

Noble H. W., Carmichael A. F. and Rankine D. M. (1962) Electron-microscopy of human developing dentine. *Arch. Oral Biol.* **7**, 395.

Nylen M. U. and Scott D. B. (1958) *An Electron Microscopic Study of the Early Stages of Dentinogenesis*. Pub. 613, U.S. Public Health Service, Washington, D. C., U.S. Government Printing Office.

Osborn J. W. (1974) The relationship between prisms and enamel tubules in the teeth of *Didelphis marsupialis*. *Arch. Oral Biol.* **19**, 835.

Osborn J. W. (1967) A mechanistic view of dentinogenesis and its relation to the curvatures of the processes of the odontoblasts. *Arch. Oral Biol.* **12**, 275.

Reith E. J. (1968) Collagen formation in developing molar teeth of rats. *J. Ultrastruct. Res.* **21**, 383.

Sisca R. F. and Provenza D. V. (1972) Initial dentine formation in human deciduous teeth. An electron microscope study. *Calc. Tiss. Res.* **9**, 1.

Stanley H. R., White C. L. and McCray L. (1966) The rate of tertiary (reparative) dentine formation in the human tooth. *Oral Surg.* **21**, 180.

Symons, N. B. B. (1956) The development of the fibres of the dentine matrix. *Br. Dent. J.* **101**, 252.

Takuma S. and Nagai N. (1971) Ultrastructure of rat odontoblasts in various stages of their development and maturation. *Arch. Oral Biol.* **16**, 993.

Ten Cate A. R. (1968) Current concepts and problems of dentinogenesis. In: Symons N. B. B. (ed.), *Dentine and Pulp*. Edinburgh, Livingstone, p. 9.

Ten Cate A. R. (1978) A fine structural study of coronal and root dentinogenesis in the mouse: observations on the so-called 'von Korff fibres' and their contribution to mantle dentine. *J. Anat. (Lond.)*, **125**, 183.

Ten Cate A. R., Melcher A. H., Pudy G. et al. (1970) The non-fibrous nature of the von Korff fibres in developing dentine. A light and electron microscopic study. *Anat. Rec.* **168**, 491.

Weidenreich F. (1925) Uber den Bau die Entwicklung des Zahnbeins in der Reihe der Wirbeltiere. *Ergebnisse der Anatomie und Entwicklungsgeschichte* **76**, 218.

Whittacker D. K. and Adams D. (1972) Electron microscopic studies on von Korff fibres in the human developing tooth. *Anat. Rec.* **174**, 175.

Yoshiki S. and Kurahashi Y. (1971) A light and electron microscopic study of alkaline phosphatase activity in the early stages of dentinogenesis in the young rat. *Arch. Oral Biol.* **16**, 1143.

CHAPTER 13

THE DENTINE PULP COMPLEX

The formation of dentine has been described as a function of the dental papilla. The dental papilla, or *dental pulp* as it is called when eventually it matures, is also responsible for the maintenance of dentine and it is therefore good practice to consider dentine and pulp as a single complex rather than two separate tissues as is usually the case. *Primary physiological dentine* is that dentine laid down rapidly during tooth development and which is completed with the formation of the apical foramen; *secondary physiological dentine* is that dentine laid down on the pulpal walls at very much slower rates after the normal anatomy of the tooth has been established. Its structure is essentially the same as the primary dentine from which it is demarcated by a resting line. It is properly regarded as physiological dentine as it is laid down in teeth which fail to erupt and therefore is not formed in response to external stimuli. Tertiary or *reparative dentine* is that dentine formed in response to some external stimulus and its structure may vary considerably depending upon the nature and degree of the stimulus. The structure of primary dentine is generally well described in standard texts and is not repeated here. Instead, only facets of dentinal structure not understood or still debatable are presented. In describing primary dentine several different distinctions are made, such as mantle dentine, circumpulpal dentine (divided into peritubular dentine and intertubular dentine) and interglobular dentine. Each will be discussed in turn.

Mantle Dentine

Mantle dentine is a layer of dentine immediately beneath the enamel in the crown and the cement in the root and is the first-formed dentine laid down by the newly differentiated odontoblast. The large fibre bundles in the collagenous matrix of mantle dentine are its main distinguishing feature. Probably because of its fibrous component mantle dentine is slightly less mineralized than the circumpulpal dentine. The development of mantle dentine has been described and the difference in fibre orientation found in root and crown mantle dentine (*see* Chapter 12). It used to be thought that the large fibres of mantle dentine were von Korff fibres (developed in the pulp) but this, too, has been discounted.

Circumpulpal Dentine

Circumpulpal dentine comprises the remainder of the primary dentine and has an organic matrix made up of much finer collagen fibrils arranged as a random network in a plane at right angles to the tubules. Circumpulpal dentine is further subdivided into intertubular dentine and peritubular dentine, the distinction being the existence of a collar of more highly mineralized dentine immediately surrounding each dentinal tubule. Peritubular dentine contains few, if any, collagen fibrils and its matrix contains glycosaminoglycans which are secreted via the odontoblast process. It has been suggested that the peritubular dentine is separated from the tubular contents by a limiting 'membrane' which is seen as an electron-dense structure. Its composition has yet to be determined. The odontoblast process in the tubule is separated from this limiting membrane by a periodontoblastic space which is occasionally occupied by thick non-mineralized collagen fibres. An unresolved problem which has not been properly studied is the formation of sclerotic (transparent) dentine which is supposed to be an extension of peritubular dentine into both the tubules and perhaps the intertubular area.

Interglobular Dentine

Interglobular dentine is not really a distinct form of dentine but discrete areas of circumpulpal dentine which have failed to mineralize. The term 'interglobular dentine' is used as the boundaries of these areas are curved and indicate the peripheries of globules which have failed to coalesce. An interesting feature is that, although dentinal tubules run interruptedly through these areas, peritubular dentine is absent. This suggests some correlation between peritubular dentine formation and the presence of mineralized dentine but this point has not been studied.

The Odontoblast

The cell associated with both the formation and maintenance of dentine is the odontoblast which has its cell body situated in the pulp. In the mature tooth the morphology of the odontoblast may vary considerably, ranging from columnar to almost squamous in shape and which reflects the functional activity of the cell. A point worth making is that most descriptions of odontoblasts, especially at the ultrastructural level, describe them in an actively secreting phase. The few ultrastructural descriptions of mature odontoblasts indicate that these cells have a much reduced organelle complement reflecting their maintenance function, but it should not be forgotten this cell has the potential to resume its secretory function when appropriately stimulated.

A key issue currently being discussed and one of great importance is the extent of the odontoblast process within the dentinal tubules. Until about 10 years ago few questioned that the process extended through the dentine as far as the amelodentinal junction. Then a scanning electron microscopic study on human premolar teeth reported that the odontoblast cell process extended no more than 0·7mm into the dentine. This report, naturally, prompted a flurry of further investigations seeking to confirm or deny this observation and all reports since that time using either the scanning or transmission electron microscope have confirmed the story. Put another way, no study in the past 10 years has been able to demonstrate the presence of an odontoblast process in dentinal tubules in the outer two-thirds of circumpulpal dentine. Even so, examination of dentine with a light microscope and sometimes with the scanning electron microscope still seems to indicate the presence of a cytoplasmic extension of the odontoblast in the outer dentine, but an explanation for this discrepancy has recently been proposed. With the electron microscope a limiting membrane has been described lining the tubule wall (*Fig. 13.1*). Its

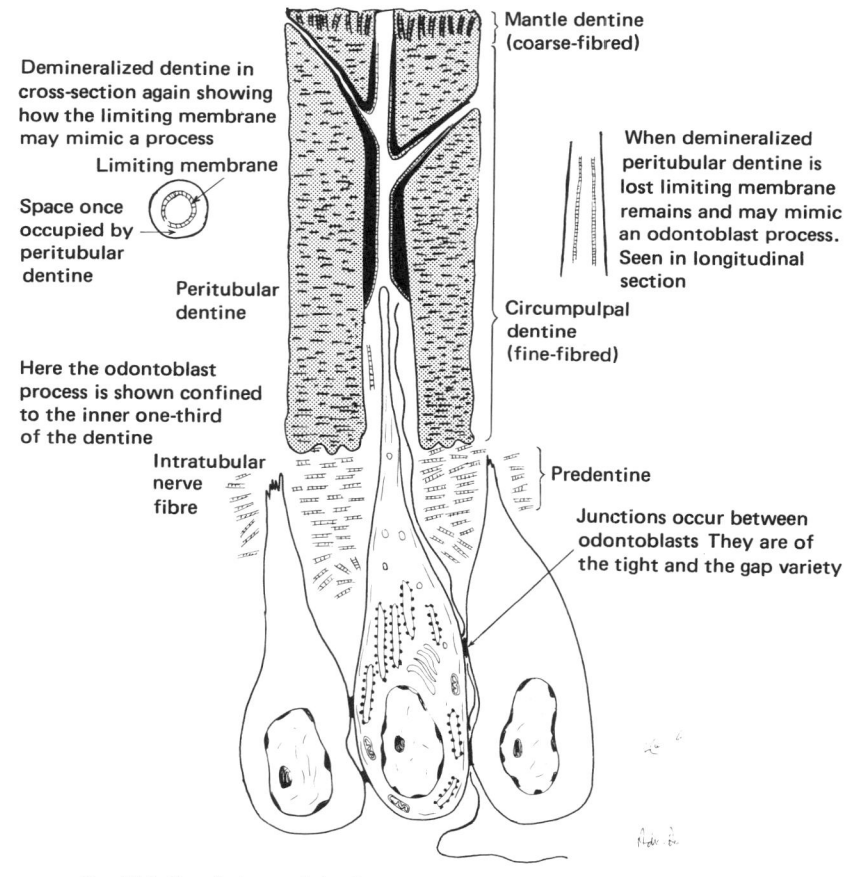

Fig. 13.1. Key features of dentine.

composition is not known but with the electron microscope it appears as an electron-dense structure which persists after demineralization removes the peritubular dentine and then mimics a process which can be seen with the light microscope and the scanning electron microscope which is only capable of demonstrating surface structures. But it is also possible that in some tubules odontoblast processes do persist and to settle the issue some form of quantitation is required.

However, until there is a clear demonstration of a cytoplasmic process in outer dentine it must be assumed that most odontoblast processes terminate in the inner one-third of the dentine. This assumption has implications in terms of dentine–pulp response to external stimuli and especially cavity preparation. For example, shallow cavity preparation was previously assumed only to damage the odontoblast process marginally so that repair took place and the cell recovered and laid down reparative dentine. Clearly shallow cavity preparation need not, and does not, sever the odontoblast process. It is only when deep cavities are cut involving the inner third of the dentine that the odontoblast process is severed and there is some preliminary evidence that when this occurs the odontoblast degenerates. For repair to occur in this circumstance new odontoblasts must therefore differentiate from undifferentiated cells in the dental pulp.

Granular Layer of Tomes

Within the subsurface of the root dentine is the granular layer of Tomes. Previously it was suggested that the granules consisted of minute interglobular spaces. However, the granules of the Tomes layer do not behave in the same way as interglobular dentine when viewed with either transmitted or incident light. The change in the optical properties of the granules of the Tomes layer when viewed first in transmitted and then in incident light indicates that the granules are true spaces. Yet when the Tomes granular layer is examined with the electron microscope no spaces are demonstrable. It has been suggested that the 'spaces' are produced by random looping of dentinal tubules (*Fig. 13.2*) in the first-formed root dentine.

Outside the Tomes granular layer a thin structureless hyaline layer can frequently be seen in ground sections and recent information indicates that this layer, although appearing to be dentine, may in fact be an epithelial cement (Chapter 17).

Thus, in summary, dentine is the mineralized component of the dentine–pulp complex. It is therefore mineralized connective tissue. It is characterized by being permeated by dentinal tubules which contain, in their inner third, protoplasmic extensions of the dentine-forming cells, the odontoblasts, which line the pulp–dentine interface. A perception of how tubular dentine is may be gained by realizing that some 30 000–70 000 tubules exist per mm^2 at the pulpal surface. Thus, dentine is porous and it

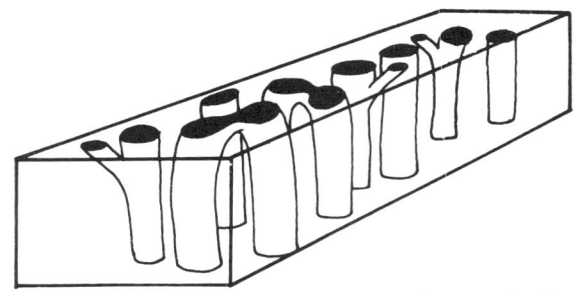

Fig. 13.2. The Tomes granular layer may represent the cut ends of branching and bending tubules.

has been estimated that in mid-dentine the total cross-sectional area of a square millimetre occupied by tubule is equivalent to a single tubule 0·3 mm in diameter—which makes dentine very porous indeed.

The pulpal component of the complex is a loosely arranged connective tissue which is responsible for its viability and hence the behaviour of the complex and its histology generally conforms to that of any other loose connective tissue.

Repair

Of particular interest is the repair response of the complex. If damage to the dentine component is such that it does not result in the death of the odontoblast, this cell is capable of initiating changes either within the dentine by introducing sclerosis or by laying down additional dentine (reparative or tertiary dentine). If, on the other hand, death of the odontoblast occurs by cavity preparation extending to the inner third of the dentine, how is repair of the complex affected? Clearly new odontoblasts are needed to lay down reparative dentine and new odontoblasts do indeed differentiate from the pulp. This presents somewhat of a conundrum because odontoblasts originally differentiated under the organizing influence of epithelial cells of either the inner dental epithelium or the root sheath (*see* Chapter 6) and, as no epithelial cells are present in the mature pulp, evidence was sought for the division of undamaged odontoblasts as a source of replacement odontoblasts. No such evidence has yet been forthcoming and, instead, findings indicate that new odontoblasts differentiate in the absence of epithelial cells from the fibroblasts of the papilla and from undifferentiated perivascular cells. This source is the same as that for reparative fibroblasts producing scar tissue in other connective tissues.

CHAPTER 14

DENTINE SENSITIVITY

The mechanism of dentine sensitivity is one of the most intriguing problems of dental histology and physiology. From common experience, most readers would not dispute that dentine is sensitive. This seems to imply the presence of nerve elements within the dentine but the majority of the nerve endings appear to be located within the pulp. It must also be remembered that histological studies alone cannot explain the mechanism of dentine sensitivity. All these can do is demonstrate a neuroanatomical pathway associated with dentine sensitivity.

Three possibilities exist which could explain the sensitivity of dentine. First, that the dentine is indeed innervated; second, that the odontoblast process and cell body have a special sensory function and are connected to a more normal neuroanatomical pathway starting in the pulp; third, the receptors associated with dentine sensitivity are located within the pulp but are capable of detecting local changes conducted mechanically through the thickness of the dentine (*Fig. 14.1*). Each of these possibilities will now be discussed in turn, beginning with the evidence for the innervation of dentine.

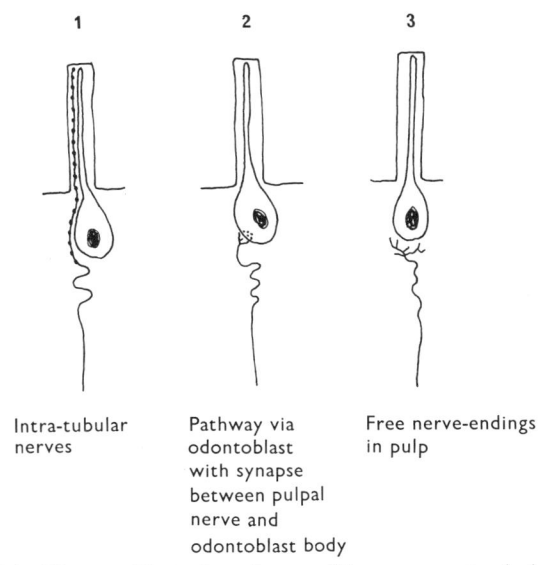

Fig. 14.1. Diagram illustrating the possible neuro-anatomical pathways associated with dentine sensitivity.

109

Innervation

No dispute exists about the presence of nerve trunks within the pulp. These can readily be demonstrated in several ways. Nor is there much dispute that these nerve trunks spread from the plexus of Raschkow beneath the odontoblasts. The disputed point is whether or not finer nerve elements enter the dentine tubules and run as far as the enamel–dentine junction. Careful and controlled histological studies have shown that nerve fibres leave the plexus of Raschkow, pass into the predentine as a loop, and pass out again to rejoin the plexus; also, what is more important, some nerve fibres enter dentinal tubules (*Fig. 14.2*). This intratubular location was first demonstrated by light microscopy and confirmed by electron microscopy and experimental autoradiographic techniques where tritiated proline was injected into the trigeminal ganglion and later demonstrated in dentinal nerves.

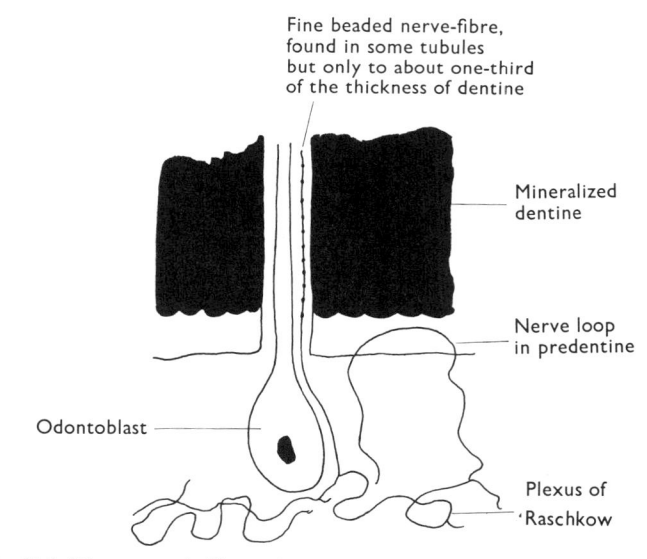

Fig. 14.2. Diagrammatic illustration of the location of nerves in dentine.

It is now clear that these intratubular nerves pass no further than 100 μm into the dentine; previous objections based on the supposition that inadequate fixation prevented their demonstration deeper in the dentine have been overcome. Furthermore, there are significant regional differences in their distribution. Thus, in human premolars in the predentine, at the mineralizing front and in mineralized dentine covering the pulpal horns the nerves are found in 27, 11 and 8 per cent of the tubules respectively, indicating a major reduction in tubular nerves within mineralized dentine. In the remainder of the crown dentine the figures are 14, 6 and 2 per cent. In root dentine no nerves occur in the tubules of mineralized dentine, although some may be found at the pulpal face of predentine, especially where the odontoblastic processes enter the predentine. The density of intratubular nerves also varies and can, in some instances, be as high as one in every second tubule in discrete areas. Considering the sensitivity of human dentine, however, remarkably few dentinal tubules appear to contain nerves and, what is more significant, newly erupted teeth do not appear to contain intradentinal nerves, despite the fact that they are sensitive.

Those nerve fibres which do enter dentinal tubules are identified in electron microscope studies by the mitochondria and vesicles which they contain. Paradoxically, these features suggest, not that the nerve fibre is monitoring changes in its environment, but rather that it is affecting the activity of the adjacent odontoblast process. This view, that the nerve fibres in dentinal tubules are motor rather than sensory nerves, receives support from the demonstration of adrenergic activity in the dentine. In other words, the nerves may be motor sympathetic terminals rather than sensory branchial receptors. However, the adrenergic activity of the dentine is not affected by cutting the cervical sympathetic chain. Had this operation abolished the adrenergic activity, it would have proved conclusively that the nerves in dentine were from the autonomic part of the nervous system with neurotrophic and metabolic supportive functions. The problem remains to be solved. During the development of the tooth it is known that 'pioneer' nerve fibres invade the dental papilla at the bell stage of development and that these fibres follow the path of the blood vessels. However, the ramification of nerves which forms the plexus of Raschkow is not established until root formation is complete. This means that the nerve fibres must grow towards the dentine if its innervation is to be established. The growing nerve tip approaching the predentine can find itself in one of two situations. It can by chance abut against the opening of the dentine tubule and pass into the lumen of the tubule, between the tubule wall and the odontoblast process. It is easy to conceive that such a growing tip pushes its way along the tubule until it meets the surface of the peritubular dentine when its extension ceases (*Fig. 14.3*). This would explain why intratubular nerve fibres are only found for a limited distance within the dentine and also why only a proportion of tubules contain them, their distribution depending on chance. The alternative situation is that a growing nerve fibre may not enter a dentine tubule but abut against the predentine surface. In this event, the growing tip will retract slightly and readvance at a different angle (*Fig. 14.4*). A succession of such steps would result in the looping of the nerve fibre, and such loops could be caught up in the forming dentine.

It is thus fair to say that there is little doubt that mineralized dentine is innervated, but it is another question whether the presence of these few

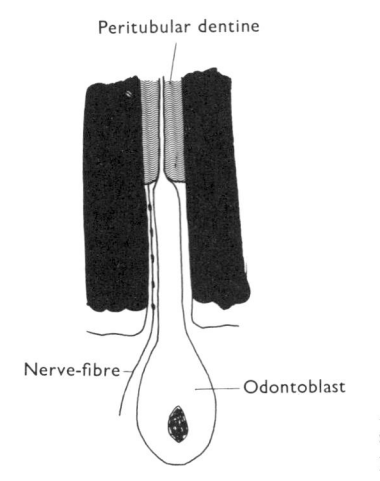

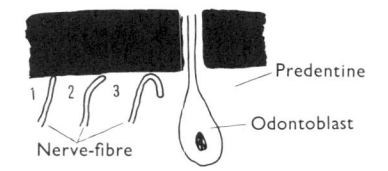

Fig. 14.4. Diagram showing how an intratubular nerve fibre might be restricted by the peritubular dentine.

Fig. 14.3. Diagram to illustrate three successive steps in the formation of a predentine nerve loop.

nerve fibres significantly influences the sensitivity of dentine. The histological demonstration of neural elements in dentine fails to explain the suggested hypersensitivity of the enamel–dentine junction or the sensitivity of newly erupted teeth.

Odontoblast Transmission

We must now discuss the evidence for considering the odontoblast as a cell capable of transmitting a stimulus in a way that is comparable to a nerve. Such a hypothesis seems to require, first, that some form of impulse is propagated down an odontoblast and, second, the presence of a functional connection between the odontoblasts and those nerve endings which continue to propagate the impulse. This functional connection may or may not be a synapse.

In support of this it was at one time reported that acetylcholinesterase was present adjacent to the bodies and processes of the odontoblasts. This enzyme is typically found in association with nerves and its presence in dentine suggested an affinity between nerves and odontoblasts. Second, because odontoblasts are probably of neural crest origin it is not unreasonable to suggest that they may retain the ability of many neural crest cells (i.e. peripheral sensory nerves and postganglionic sympathetic nerves) to propagate an impulse. Third, electron microscopical studies have demonstrated a seemingly close functional relationship between nerve endings and the processes of odontoblasts and odontoblast cell bodies. Finally, the fact that odontoblast processes branch profusely in the region of the enamel dentine junction could explain the reported hypersensitivity of the enamel–dentine junction on the basis of a summation phenomenon.

However, all the above findings have been either refuted or disputed. A more reliable method of assessing the presence of acetylcholinesterase has failed to demonstrate its presence in dentine at the light microscope level but a trace of possible activity has been indicated at the fine structural level. The membrane potential of odontoblasts has been measured in tissue culture (N. B. not *in vivo*) and found to be too low to take part in an excitable process but, again, this observation has recently been challenged. The question of a junction between odontoblast and neural elements is clearly crucial to the hypothesis and warrants detailed exploration. The first point that should be made, however, is that even if a 'synaptic' junction can be proved it does not settle the issue of dentine sensitivity for it still is necessary to determine whether the nerve is afferent or efferent. It has already been indicated that whenever neural elements and the odontoblast (either cell body or process) come into close apposition and exhibit the morphological features of a synapse, the vesicular and mitochondrial components are always in the neural element which would indicate transduction from neurone to odontoblast.

Gap junctions, specialization of cell membranes tailored for intercellular communications, can be found between adjacent odontoblasts, and perhaps between nerve axons and odontoblasts, and in the presence of such junctions could explain the diffuseness of dental pain again on the basis of a summation of many odontoblasts. The key, though, is the clear identification of a gap junction and/or synapse between nerve and odontoblast which has not yet been done.

Hydrodynamic Theory

If the odontoblast process does not propagate an electrical impulse, it remains to explain how a stimulus applied to the largely nerve-free dentine can be transmitted to the nerve endings deep within the tooth. The possibility exists of a purely physical rather than biological transmission of the stimulus. For example, it has been suggested that temperature changes at the surface of a tooth could be physically transmitted, by conduction, through the mineralized dentine to the pulp. But carefully timed responses to pain-producing stimuli have indicated that the speed of transmission is far greater than could be predicted by simple conduction. The times were closely related to those which could be predicted if the stimulus caused the movement of fluid through the dentine due to surface contractions and expansions consequent on temperature changes.

This is a part of the evidence which suggests that fluid movements in the dentine could be responsible for evoking the initiation of impulses from nerve endings. It has not been possible to test this directly; experiments have so far been limited to determining first whether fluid can move through dentine and second whether pain is evoked when the fluid can be presumed to have moved.

The rapid movement of fluid through dentine has now been demonstrated many times *in vitro*. A capillary is sealed to the root of a tooth from which the pulp has been removed (*Fig. 14.5*). The excavated pulp and capillary are filled with saline. A cavity is cut into the dentine. If solutions of high osmotic pressure (for instance, sugar solutions) are applied to the cut surface of the dentine, fluid is rapidly sucked through the capillary. Still greater movements are produced by drying the dentine with a blast of air or by cutting the dentine with a drill.

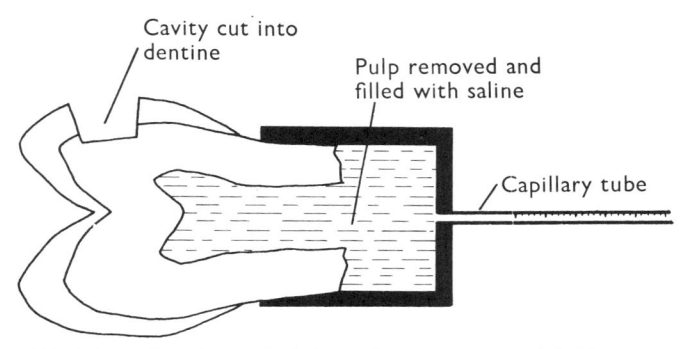

Fig. 14.5. Illustrating the method by which movements of fluid through dentine have been measured.

It can be shown that each of the above operations causes pain *in vivo* and that the amount of pain is roughly proportional to the fluid movement observed *in vitro*. It is tentatively concluded that the movement of fluid through dentine causes stimulation of nerve endings either in the pulp or in the dentine. The fluid which moves may be accommodated in either the periodontoblastic space or the process of the odontoblast, or both. In any event it is probably the eventual movement of interstitial fluid in the pulp which would initiate the stimulation of the nerve fibres. This is the basis of the suggestion that there is a hydrodynamic transmission of pain-producing stimuli, but a real problem here is that *in vitro* water causes fluid movement but *in vivo* does not cause pain when applied to exposed dentine.

All the current theories of dentine sensitivity have now been discussed. Many questions still remain. For example, it could be that stimuli applied to dentine cause pain by more than one mechanism such as electrical and thermal stimuli directly affecting pulpal nerves, whereas others may involve fluid movements in the tubules and the pulp.

DENTINE SENSITIVITY

The Diffuse Response

Another intriguing question concerning dentine sensitivity is the diffuseness of the pain response. There are several anatomical bases for this, whatever the true mechanism of dentine sensitivity. First is the branching of dentinal tubules close to the amelo-dentinal junction. This branching provides a greater number of odontoblast processes or tubules per unit area for either the odontoblast transmitter or hydrodynamic theories. Second is the demonstrated occurrence of numerous gap junctions between odontoblasts which could lead to potentiation of a stimulus applied to a single odontoblast. Third is the fact that many nerves lose their myelin sheathes in the pulp, with axon-to-axon contact occurring. Finally, it is known from retrograde labelling studies (which apply a marker to exposed pulps to be picked up by local neural elements and transported centrally) that the representation of pulpal neurones is distributed throughout the trigeminal nucleus. Each of these features could provide the anatomical basis for the diffuseness of dental pain.

Why is Dentine Sensitive?

If dentine is sensitive and pain is the only result of any successful stimulus, the painful sensation must have some selective advantage in terms of evolution. But it is remarkably difficult to conceive any advantage in this painful response. Potentially noxious excesses of temperature and pressure are monitored by the oral mucosa and periodontal ligament, tissues which are far more easily damaged than dentine. One possible answer is that when dentine has been worn away by attrition and there is no secondary dentine sealing the pulp, pain might be felt. This would encourage mastication of food in another part of the mouth until secondary dentine had been deposited.

Another solution to this problem suggests that dentine might act like an enormous pressure receptor, detecting the direction and amount of force applied to the individual cusps of teeth (nerves supplying the periodontal ligament can only integrate the direction and amount of force applied to every cusp on the tooth). When a cusp is compressed, fluid could be squeezed down dentinal tubules initiating a patterned response from the pulpal afferent nerve fibres which supply that cusp. This patterned response could be interpreted within the central nervous system as the direction and amount of pressure applied to a tooth cusp.

The above explanation needs to be compared with the generally accepted view that the movement of fluid down dentinal tubules evokes a sensation of pain in man (and all animals?). It is very unlikely that stimuli such as extremes of temperature, desiccation and osmosis are ever received by a normal dentition. The only naturally applied stimulus would be pressure. If pressure is applied to a tooth, it seems inevitable that periodontal afferents would be stimulated. Therefore (almost) without exception, whenever fluid is moved down dentinal tubules by pressure applied to the cusp of a tooth (thereby stimulating pulpal afferents), periodontal afferents are simultaneously stimulated. In this situation, the discharge of pulpal efferents is not interpreted as pain. However, in an abnormal experimental situation it is possible to move large volumes of fluid down dentinal tubules (e.g. by applying solutions of high osmotic pressure) without stimulating periodontal afferents. Such large fluid movements would normally be associated with very heavy pressure on the tooth. In the absence of this expected sensation of pressure it is possible that the central nervous system interprets the abnormal isolated activity of pulpal afferents as a painful sensation.

It could equally be argued that dentine sensitivity is purely fortuitous. So much of the pattern of innervation of the pulp dentine complex can be attributed to chance innervation based on the known characteristics of growing nerve fibres. If it is supposed that the prime requirement for innervation of the dental apparatus is the innervation of supporting tissues, which are known to be essential for providing information as to tooth contact and jaw position, it can be postulated that some pioneer nerve fibres destined for the ligament enter the dental papilla. Once in the papilla they ramify, as already described in this chapter, as in the plexus of Rashkow and in some tubules.

Then, if dentine sensitivity is explained by direct innervation of dentine or the hydrodynamic theory, both demand the presence of tubules in dentine. In other words, if dentine were not tubular would it be sensitive? It should be worth while to examine the sensitivity of other dentines which are non-tubular, such as vaso-dentine, which represents a complex folding of the pulp dentine interface. These forms of dentine and, of course, tubular dentine represent anatomical configurations to provide proper nutrition of the dentine matrix, and it is just possible that tubular dentine may only coincidentally provide the needed anatomical basis for dentine sensitivity.

REFERENCES AND FURTHER READING

Anderson D. J., Matthews B. and Goretta C. (1967) Fluid flow through human dentine. *Arch. Oral Biol.* **12**, 209.

Anderson D. J. and Ronning G. A. (1962) Dye diffusion in human dentine. *Arch. Oral Biol.* **7**, 505.

Anderson D. J. and Ronning G. A. (1962) Osmotic excitants of pain in human dentine *Arch. Oral Biol.* **7**, 513.

Brannstrom M. (1966) Sensitivity of dentine. *Oral Surg.* **21**, 517.

Brannstrom M. and Astrom A. (1972) The hydrodynamics of the dentine; its possible relationship to dentinal pain. *Int. Dent. J.* **22**, 219.

Brannstrom M. and Johnson G. (1970) Movements of the dentine and pulp liquids on application of thermal stimuli. An *in vitro* study. *Acta Odont. Scand.* **28**, No. 1, p. 59.

Brannstrom M., Johnson G. and Linden L.-A. (1969) Fluid flow and pain response in the dentine produced by hydrostatic pressure. *Odontologisk Revy* **20**, 1.

Brannstrom M. and Lind P. O. (1965) Pulpal response to early dental caries. *J. Dent. Res.* **44**, No. 5, p. 1045.

Brannstrom M., Linden, L.-A. and Johnson G. (1968) Movement of dentinal and pulpal fluid caused by clinical procedures. *J. Dent. Res.* **47**, No. 5, p. 679.

Byers M. R. and Matthews B. (1981) Autoradiographic demonstration of ipsilateral and contralateral sensory nerve endings in cat dentine, pulp and periodontium. *Anat. Rec.* **201**, 249.

Corpron R. E. and Avery J. K. (1973) The ultrastructure of intradental nerves in developing mouse molars. *Anat. Rec.* **175**(3), 585.

Dahl E. and Mjor I. A. (1973) The structure and distribution of nerves in the pulp–dentine organ. *Acta Odont. Scand.* **31**, 349.

Fearnhead R. W. (1957) Histological evidence for the innervation of human dentine. *J. Anat.* **91**, 267.

Fearnhead R. W. (1963) The histological demonstration of nerve fibers in human dentine. In: Anderson D. J. (ed.), *Sensory Mechanisms in Dentine*. Oxford, Pergamon Press.

Frank R. M. (1968) Attachment sites between the odontoblast process and the intradental nerve fibre. *Arch. Oral Biol.* **13**, 833.

Harris R. and Griffin C. J. (1968) Fine structure of nerve endings in the human dental pulp. *Arch. Oral Biol.* **13**, 773.

Holland G. R. (1976) The extent of the odontoblast process in the cat. *J. Anat.* **121**, No. 1, p. 133.

Johnson G. and Brannstrom M. (1974) The sensitivity of dentine changes in relation to conditions at exposed tubule apertures. *Acta Odont. Scand.* **32**, 29.

Johnson G. and Brannstrom M. (1971) Pain reaction to cold stimulus in teeth with experimental fillings. *Acta Odont. Scand.* **29**, 639.

Linden L.-A. and Brannstrom M. (1967) Fluid movements in dentine and pulp. An *in vitro* study of flow produced by chemical solutions on exposed dentine. *Odontologisk Revy* **18**, No. 3, p. 227.

Pohto P. and Antila R. (1968) Acetylcholinesterase and noradrenaline in the nerves of mammalian dental pulps. *Acta Odont. Scand.* **26**, No. 6, p. 641.

Powers, M. M. (1952) The staining of nerve fibers in teeth. *J. Dent. Res.* **31**, 383.

CHAPTER 15

AMELOGENESIS

Although enamel is ectodermal in origin, as opposed to mesodermal, and although it contains an extremely high proportion of inorganic material (96 per cent by weight), its formation is fundamentally similar to that of the other mineralized tissues of the body; a cellular layer produces a matrix which is subsequently mineralized with hydroxyapatite.

At the bell stage of tooth development, when the crown pattern of the tooth is being determined, the base of the enamel organ consists of a single layer of short columnar cells, the inner dental epithelium (*Fig. 15.1*). The remaining tissues of the dental organ are the stratum intermedium, stellate reticulum, and the outer dental epithelium. At the time the odontoblasts begin their path towards differentiation, the cells of the inner dental epithelium increase in length, their cytoplasm accumulates an increasing amount of 'smooth' and 'rough' endoplasmic reticulum and free ribosomes, and their mitochondria move to the end of the cell nearest the stratum intermedium (*Fig. 15.2*). These changes prepare for the production of enamel for which purpose the stratum intermedium and the inner dental epithelium can be regarded as a single functional unit. Alkaline phosphatase is found exclusively in the stratum intermedium during enamel matrix formation, while the inner dental epithelium is rich in RNA and oxidative enzymes. These histochemical features parallel those found in the cells forming other hard tissues.

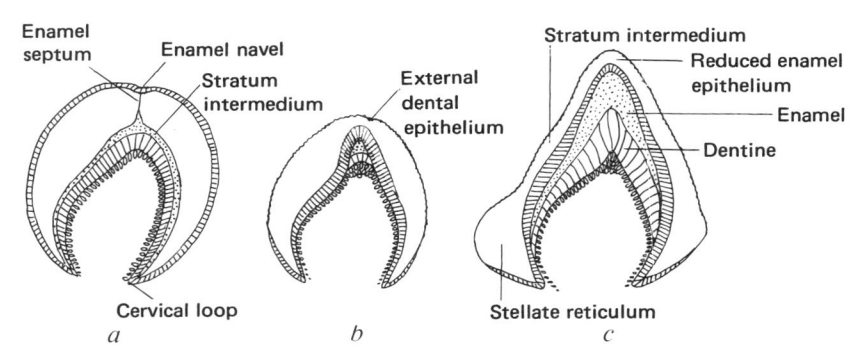

Fig. 15.1. Just before amelogenesis the stellate reticulum separates the stratum intermedium from the internal enamel epithelium (*a*). The stellate reticulum collapses opposite the region where amelogenesis begins (*b*) and continues to collapse around the sides of the tooth as amelogenesis spreads away from the cusp tip (*c*).

AMELOGENESIS

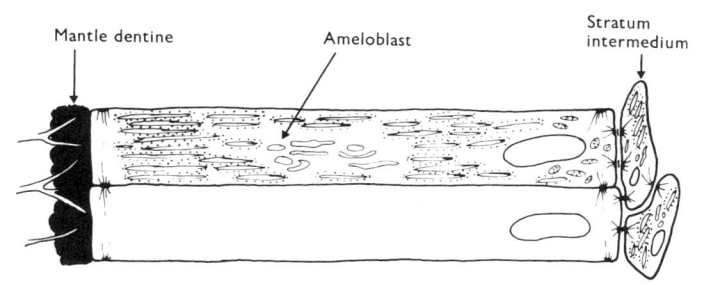

Fig. 15.2. A preameloblast, just before amelogenesis begins.

DIFFERENTIATION OF AMELOBLASTS

The point has been made that the formative cells of the other hard tissues differentiate in regions of high vascularity. This is not the case for the inner dental epithelium. These cells differentiate into functional ameloblasts in a relatively avascular situation.

From the time at which a tooth bud is initiated it seems that the cells of the inner dental epithelium have become programmed towards their function of developing the enamel. Their cell division, change of polarity, manufacture of organelles, increase in size and final cessation of mitosis are described in Chapter 6. Although the pulpal cells may (or may not) control each stage in the sequence their presence adjacent to the inner dental epithelium seems essential for the continuation of the sequence (cf. mesodermal maintenance factor). The evidence for this is that if the dental organ is grown in isolation its cells regress to become a flattened epithelium.

Prior to secreting the initial enamel proteins the cells of the inner dental epithelium seem poised as they await a final induction cue. The nature of this final cue is unknown although it probably depends on a reaction to the subjacent, newly developed and mineralized first layer of dentine. Evidence for this is based on the observation in experimental situations that enamel fails to develop opposite regions where mineralized dentine is not formed.

The onset of amelogenesis is marked by the aggregation of vesicles containing stippled material at the secretory pole of the ameloblasts. The vesicles fuse with the cell membrane which now ruptures and their contents become extracellular (*Fig. 15.3*). This discharged material is the organic matrix of the first-formed enamel. It is evident, therefore, that enamel is formed by a secretory process and not by conversion of the protoplasm of the ameloblast as was once believed. The ameloblasts move outwards away from the dentine surface as more enamel matrix is

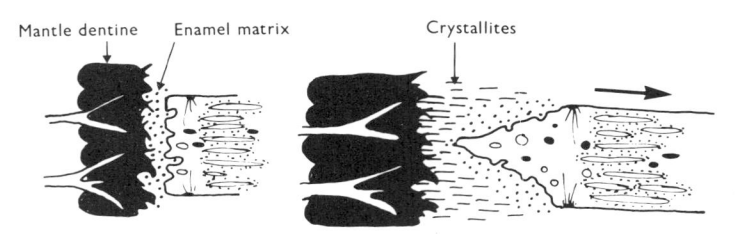

Fig. 15.3. The start of enamel matrix formation and the development of a Tomes process.

secreted. When sufficient matrix has been deposited between the secretory end of an ameloblast and the outer surface of the dentine, its cell membrane becomes pushed into the matrix as the conical Tomes process through which further matrix is secreted (*Fig. 15.3*).

Almost coincidental with this deposition of enamel matrix needle-like crystals of hydroxyapatite appear within it. Thus unlike the other hard tissues, there is no clear-cut band of organic matrix such as predentine or osteoid preceding mineralization. As enamel crystallites appear almost immediately in newly secreted enamel matrix by common usage the term 'enamel matrix' has come to be recognized as containing both organic and inorganic material. It seems likely that both the organic and the inorganic material are secreted together in the stippled vesicles (*see later*).

The ameloblasts continue moving backwards and secreting material. They are pursued by the lengthening crystals which are separated from the Tomes process by a region about 100 nm thick containing stippled material. It can safely be assumed that new crystals are constantly being initiated to replace those whose ends terminate at the sides of prisms. No matrix vesicles have been seen in developing enamel so it appears they are not required for the initiation of enamel crystals. The first crystals may grow from the 'free' ends of those already present in dentine but this is only a suggestion.

HISTOLOGY OF THE ENAMEL ORGAN

Just before amelogenesis begins the pre-ameloblasts are widely separated from a source of nutrition. On one side they are separated from pulpal vessels by mineralized dentine and on the other side a thick stellate reticulum intervenes between follicular vessels which are beginning to proliferate adjacent to the outer dental epithelium. Prior to this 'isolation' the pre-ameloblasts have been storing glycogen and this is used as a source of energy during early amelogenesis.

Amelogenesis begins at the tip of the primary (dentine) cusp and spreads down its sides. This is rapidly followed by a 'collapse' of the stellate reticulum adjacent to areas of amelogenesis thereby bringing the ameloblasts and stratum intermedium in contact with the outer dental epithelium (*Fig. 15.1b*). The fate of the cells of the stellate reticulum is not understood. During early enamel formation the cuspal cells may be mechanically displaced around the sides of the tooth leading to the slight convex bulge of the inner dental epithelium towards the pulp. In human incisors there is a consistently larger volume of stellate reticulum on the lingual surfaces. This discrepancy is maintained as the stellate reticulum steadily shrinks while amelogenesis is spreading towards what will ultimately be the cervical margin. Finally, the stellate reticulum disappears entirely.

The outer dental epithelium originally consists of cuboidal cells. With the onset of amelogenesis they become flattened and the whole surface corrugated (*Fig. 15.1b*). These changes together with the appearance of numerous capillaries adjacent to the surface of the dental organ are taken to indicate an improvement in the capacity of the outer dental epithelium to absorb nutrients required for amelogenesis and to expel related waste products.

All the cells of the dental organ are connected by desmosomes. The outer dental epithelium is connected to a basal lamina, which separates it from the dental follicle, by hemi-desmosomes. The cells contain a little rough-surfaced endoplasmic reticulum (RER) and Golgi material. The stellate reticulum cells contain Golgi material (associated with the formation and ultimate secretion of proteoglycans and glycoproteins). They also have microvilli on their plasma membranes. The stratum intermedium contains both RER (therefore protein secreting) and Golgi material. On its surface, microvilli extend towards the ameloblasts. All the cells of the dental organ, apart from ameloblasts, contain alkaline phosphatase.

The ameloblasts (*Fig. 15.4*) are tall columnar cells about 5 μm wide and 40–50 μm long. Towards their ends the sides of adjacent ameloblasts are connected by junctional complexes (*see Fig. 2.3*) which effectively seal them together and prevent material passing between them. Along their sides they are connected by further desmosomes and gap junctions. At their proximal ends they are connected to the stratum intermedium by desmosomes and an interdigitation of microvilli from both layers.

The tonofilaments of a (proximal) terminal bar apparatus (*see Fig. 2.3.*) stretch across the proximal cytoplasm. Numerous mitochondria separate the nucleus from this web of filaments. The cytoplasm of the ameloblast is largely filled with RER. The centre of the cytoplasm distal to the nucleus contains a well-developed Golgi complex whose saccules mature towards the centre of the cell. From here membrane-bound granules can be seen and these pass towards the Tomes process. A distal terminal web associated with a distal junctional complex separates the RER from the cytoplasm of the Tomes process which contains numerous granules and vesicles. The ameloblasts seem tightly bound together and material cannot

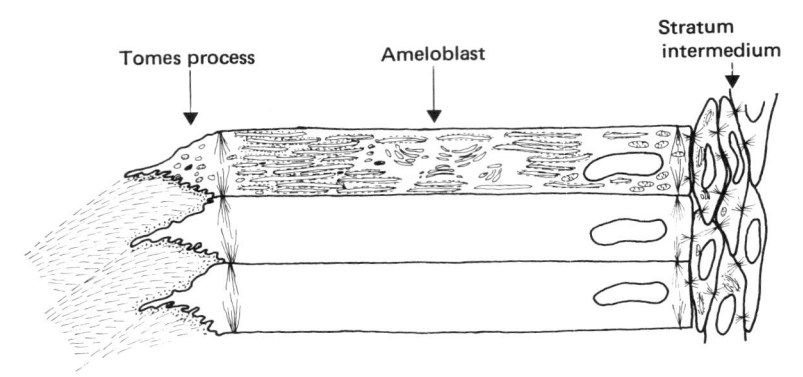

Fig. 15.4. A fully differentiated ameloblast (seen in the longitudinal plane of a tooth).

leak between the junctional complexes which tie them. Nevertheless, the ameloblasts cross each other to form criss-crossing rows of prisms (*see Fig. 16.3*).

ENAMEL MATRIX

The freshly secreted product of ameloblasts contains 65 per cent water, 20 per cent organic material as proteins; very small amounts of proteoglycans, glycosaminoglycans, citrate and lipid; and 15 per cent inorganic ions of phosphate and calcium.

The nature of the organic component is still poorly understood, the problem being related to the very small quantity present in enamel and the difficulty of isolating it for analysis.

The proteinaceous material is probably incorporated outside the ameloblast into an amorphous gel rather than an orientated assembly of fibres. Constituents of this newly secreted gel can move deeply into the developing enamel and back into later secreted material. This has been shown by following in timed series of electron micrographs the movement of different amino-acids which have been radioactively labelled, injected into an animal, and subsequently incorporated into the developing enamel (*Fig. 15.5*).

Only the proteins in enamel have been investigated in any detail, and currently two schools of thought exist as to their nature. Some believe that the ameloblast secretes a single protein, amelogenin, which has the form of an amorphous gel. This protein rapidly breaks up into smaller fragments, one fragment of which is distinctive because (1) it is highly acidic, (2) it is of relatively high molecular size (40 000D), (3) it is tightly bound to enamel crystal surfaces and (4) it occurs only in small amounts (1 per cent

AMELOGENESIS

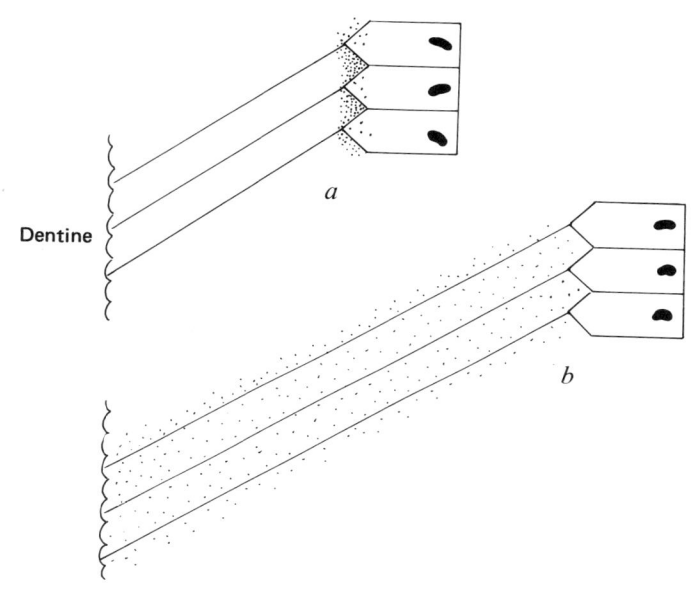

Fig. 15.5. Four hours after radioactive proline has been injected into the abdomen, sections prepared from a developing tooth show the radioactive material in a discrete band being secreted by ameloblasts (*a*). Animals killed 4 days later show that this material has spread into enamel formed before the injection and back into enamel formed after the injection (*b*).

of the protein content of the newly secreted matrix). The name 'enamelin' has been given to this protein. Others believe that enamelin and amelogenenin are distinct and separate proteins, secreted by the ameloblast and arising from different gene products. Whatever the correct interpretation, it is useful to think of enamel matrix as consisting of enamelin and amelogenins (smaller fragments of the original amelogenin). During maturation of enamel the amelogenins, which are characterized by a high proline content, are almost entirely removed from the enamel so that the amino-acid analysis of mature enamel matrix is very different from that of the first secreted protein (*Fig. 15.6*). Because enamelin is tightly bound to crystallites this protein comprises most of the residual protein in enamel.

CRYSTAL GROWTH

It has already been stated that as the ameloblasts secrete matrix and move away from the dentine, the newly developed, needle-like crystals lengthen so that only about 100 nm separates their growing ends from the surface of

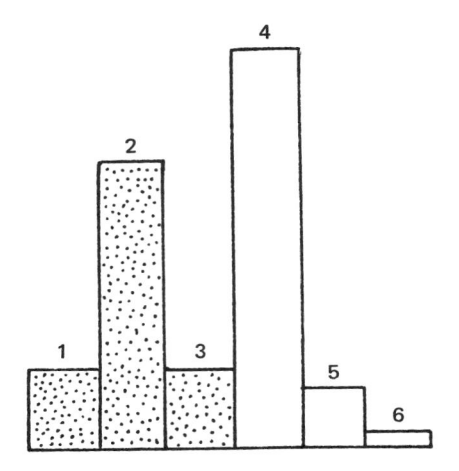

Fig. 15.6. Histogram showing the change in amino-acid composition during enamel maturation. Stippled: before maturation. The numbers represent the number of amino-acid residues per 1000 total residues. 1, Glycine 67; 2, Proline 243; 3, Histidine 63; 4, Glycine 305; 5, Proline 47; 6, Histidine 9.

the retreating Tomes processes. In cross-section the early crystals are somewhat flattened hexagons, are randomly orientated and occupy about 27 per cent of the volume of the young enamel. Later they thicken at their sides and come to occupy about 88 per cent of the volume. Their edges now almost touch and the crystals can no longer grow and maintain the hexagonal cross-section dictated by the crystal lattice of hydroxyapatite. In other words, the percentage of space occupied by the mature crystals is physically determined. It can be appreciated that were it not for the fact that the amorphous gel which surrounds the growing crystals (and from which they abstract the inorganic ions required for their growth) can be displaced it would not be possible for them to grow to the huge size which characterizes them.

MATURATION OF ENAMEL

Microradiographs indicate that the crystals do not increase in thickness at a uniform rate. After a certain period of slow increase in radio-opacity, which seems to differ between species, the enamel rapidly achieves its full mineralization. This indicates a delayed but rapid increase in crystal thickness and is known as enamel maturation. During the process inorganic ions are incorporated into the developing enamel and protein and water are lost. Enamel maturation can only be partly under cellular control (ameloblasts). A physicochemical component must also exist since the actual events of maturation take place a considerable distance away from the ameloblasts.

The maturation of human enamel prisms, for example, begins long before their associated ameloblasts have completed developing the full

AMELOGENESIS

length of the prism. In this case, the ameloblasts secrete new material and at the same time absorb the water and protein ejected or released by enamel maturing deep in the crown. From the appearance of electron micrographs of amelogenesis in the cat it has been concluded that the cervical surface of the Tomes process secretes material while its cuspal surface absorbs material, the apex of the Tomes process being the 'watershed' between secretion and absorption.

When the full length of a cuspal prism has been developed in man, approximately half of it is close to full maturation. The outer half contains only about one-third of its final mineral. The events which now take place have been most closely studied in rodent incisors. In their much thinner enamel the full thickness of matrix develops before it matures. It has been shown that the ameloblast at this time develops a brush border adjacent to the formed enamel matrix (in other words, an increase in its surface area) and that mitochondria accumulate adjacent to this brush border (*Fig. 15.7*). Activity of the enzyme acid phosphatase increases and aminopeptidase activity becomes demonstrable within the ameloblast for the

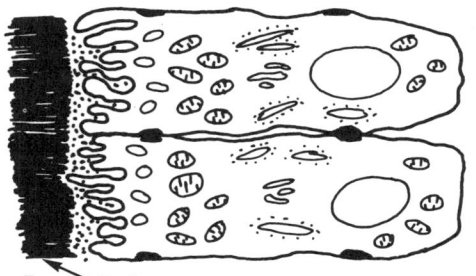

Fig. 15.7. Ameloblast at the end of amelogenesis. cf. *Fig. 15.4.*

first time. Both are catabolic enzymes prominent in osteoclasts, for example. This suggests that the ameloblasts may now be degrading material selectively removed from the enamel matrix. At the same time they are also involved with the influx of mineral salts into the changing matrix. It has already been pointed out that during enamel matrix formation the mineral salts may be passed into the matrix via the secretory vesicles. This route is no longer available with the completion of matrix formation and the most likely way that mineral salts can now pass into enamel is through the ameloblasts and across the brush border. There is evidence from other sources, such as calcium transport in the gut and in the avian shell gland, that activity of the enzyme alkaline phosphatase is required for calcium transport across membranes and it is perhaps significant that this enzyme first becomes active within the ameloblast at the time the brush border develops and indeed is associated with it.

Ameloblasts persist in a viable form up until the time of tooth eruption. There is evidence that between the completion of rapid enamel maturation and tooth eruption, which may be called the 'pre-eruptive maturation phase', important changes take place in the composition of enamel mediated by the ameloblasts. When enamel is analysed it is possible to show that gradients of concentration exist for several of its constituents. Thus the concentration of sodium, magnesium and carbonate is highest at the dentine–enamel junction and is almost halved in the surface layers of enamel. Conversely, such elements as fluoride, lead and zinc have their highest concentrations in the surface layers of enamel. These important gradients are established during the pre-eruptive phase of enamel maturation. Sodium, magnesium and carbonate incorporated into the hydroxyapatite crystal make it more soluble in water and acid while fluoride, zinc, lead and tin make it less soluble. These gradients are important in relation to caries because they all lessen the solubility of surface enamel.

PRISM FORMATION

So far, enamel formation has been described without reference to prisms. The relationship between ameloblasts and prisms is difficult to appreciate due to the problem of visualizing the process in three dimensions. This difficulty is compounded by differences in the terminology used to describe enamel structure. It all depends on whether prisms are defined as roughly circular and surrounded by an interprismatic region or keyhole-shaped and interlocking. Using the latter terminology, a prism develops within the region bounded by the apices of four Tomes processes (*Fig. 15.8b*) and is developed from four ameloblasts. If the prisms are defined as being circular, one ameloblast forms one prism and its surrounding interprismatic region (*Fig. 15.8a*).

The relationship between ameloblasts and developing prisms can be visualized by making the model given in *Fig. 15.9*. Faces 2a and 2b represent the appearance seen in a longitudinally sectioned tooth; Face 1 cuts the prisms horizontally; and Face 3 cuts them vertically.

The Longitudinal Plane (Faces 2a and 2b)

The long axis of an ameloblast is angled to the long axis of the prism it is producing. Each prism sheath is continuous with the apex of a Tomes process and corresponds with an abrupt change in the orientation of crystals. From its cuspal to its cervical edge the long axes (c-axes) of the crystals within a prism gradually deviate from parallel to the long axis of the prism to about 60° or 70° to its long axis. In this plane of section, which cuts prisms through their vertical diameter, the adjacent Tomes processes are separated by the edges of intervening ameloblasts. It can be visualized that a slightly deeper plane of section would begin to cut the Tomes processes of these intervening ameloblasts.

AMELOGENESIS

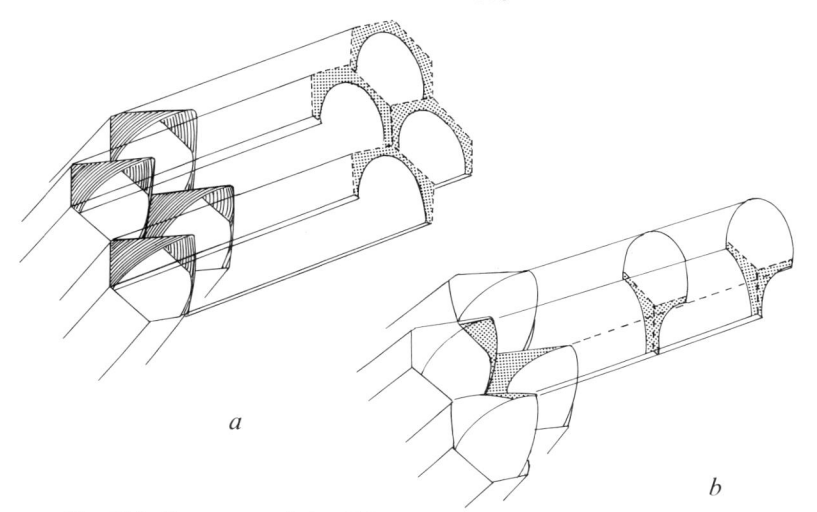

Fig. 15.8. Two ways of visualizing amelogenesis. *a*, Circular prisms surrounded by interprismatic regions (stippled) corresponding with the (shaded) cuspal borders of the Tomes processes. *b*, Keyhole-shaped prisms with their tails (stippled) developed from the cuspal surfaces of three ameloblasts (stippled) surrounding a 'valley' bordered by four ameloblasts.

The Horizontal Plane (of the Prism) (Face 1)

The prisms are in line with the ameloblasts. The Tomes processes are flattened producing what has been called a 'battlements' profile (as opposed to the 'picket fence' profile in the longitudinal plane). Prism sheaths are continuous with the corners of the battlements. Between adjacent prism sheaths the crystals funnel away from the Tomes process towards the middle of the sectioned prism.

Perpendicular to the Prism Axis (Face 3)

The interpretations of the appearance of this face cause most of the problems associated with understanding both enamel structure and amelogenesis. The actual appearance seen in ground sections of human enamel and in many electron micrographs is shown on the left of Face 3. The prism sheaths are C-shaped with their open ends facing cervically. This appearance has been interpreted in the two different ways described in Chapter 16. On the upper right side of Face 3 it can be seen that one ameloblast forms one roughly circular prism, open on its cervical side. The diagram reveals that, rather than circular, the prism is more accurately visualized as an inverted tear-drop. The tip of the tear-drop is in line with the cervical end of the cervical face of the Tomes process secreting the prism (a dotted line from ameloblast B indicates this). An interprismatic region develops around each tear-drop but is continuous with the prism so that no prism sheath separates them (left of Face 3). By following the line from the tip of the Tomes process of ameloblast B to the cuspal edge of the (bisected) prism it produces on Face 3, it can be seen that an ameloblast produces a prism and its surrounding interprismatic region. This is also shown in *Fig. 15.8*.

The relation between ameloblasts and the keyhole interpretation is shown at the bottom right of Face 3 (*Fig. 15.9*). With this interpretation, at any one time four ameloblasts are forming one prism.

The decussation of prisms is described in Chapter 16; rows of prisms cross each other in the transverse plane of the tooth. It can be seen from *Fig. 15.10* that as a prism begins to cross over two cervically adjacent prisms its tail is withdrawn and an interprismatic region develops. When the crossing is complete, two of the three ameloblasts forming the tail are replaced (13 and 23 have been replaced by 15 and 25). This text has rejected the concept of interlocking keyhole-shaped prisms in human enamel without an interprismatic region because such a region is always being developed when prisms cross each other and is also developed during early enamel formation (*see Fig. 16.1*). Furthermore, due to prism decussation, perhaps 10–20 ameloblasts are required to form each prism. In the simpler analysis proposed here, one ameloblast forms the same prism and its associated interprismatic region throughout amelogenesis.

HYPOTHESES

There are no experimental data showing how a prism is formed. The shapes of prisms vary from species to species, there being three major types (*Fig. 15.11*). Their arrangement varies from the straight prisms in most insectivores to adjacent rows of prisms crossing each other at right angles, the condition present in some rodents such as the rat and mouse. The cellular mechanisms controlling these differences are unknown. All that can be said for certain is that they are genetically determined, but this information is of little value in understanding the process of amelogenesis.

The following unified hypothesis is given here because it attempts to integrate the majority of observations.

By means of their basal mitochondria the ameloblasts draw in water and associated nutrients and raw materials from the body of the enamel organ. This raises the intracellular pressure (*Fig. 15.12b*) compressing the (potentially circular) cross-sections of ameloblasts into a hexagonal array (Face 4, *Fig. 15.9*). Clearly the only possible exit for material is from the opposite (ultimately secreting) ends of the ameloblasts; material cannot leave at the sides. When the intracellular pressure exceeds the extracellular pressure, material is secreted (*Fig. 15.12c*). This causes the extracellular

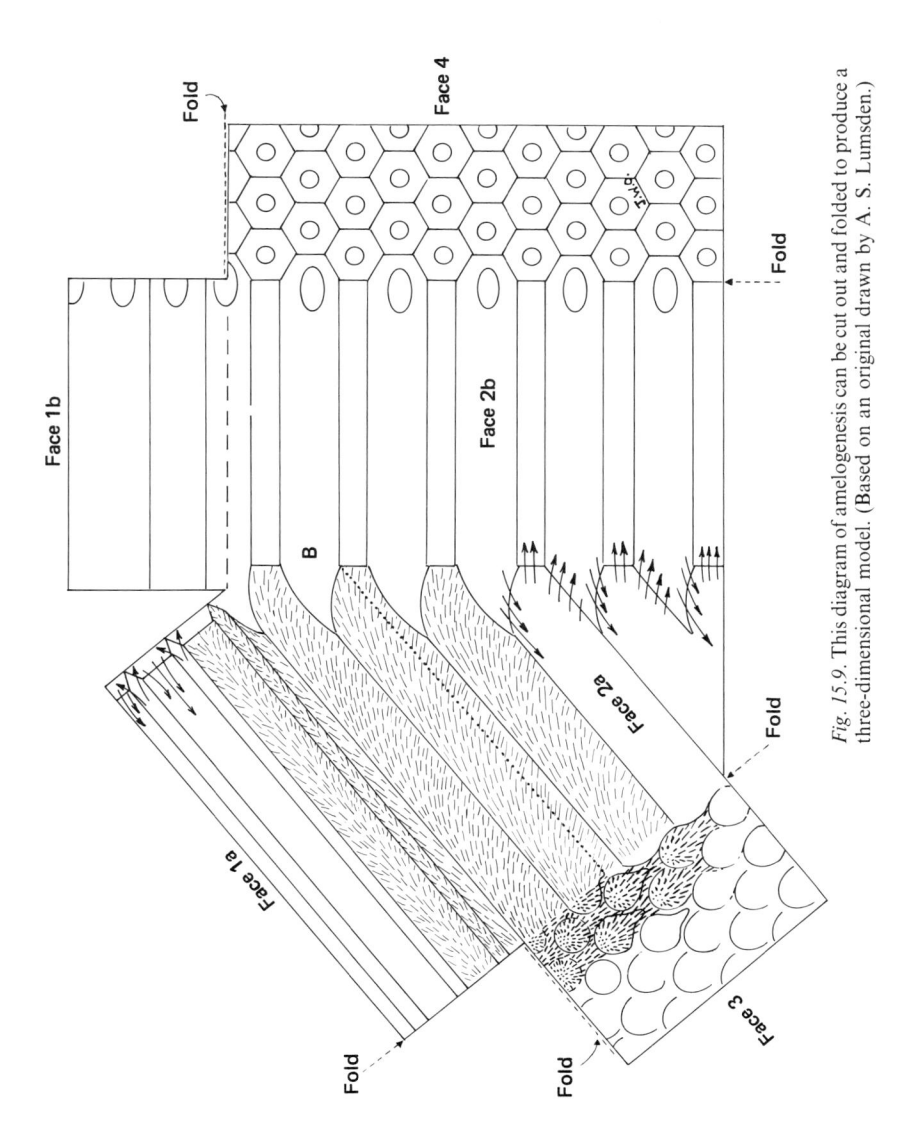

Fig. 15.9. This diagram of amelogenesis can be cut out and folded to produce a three-dimensional model. (Based on an original drawn by A. S. Lumsden.)

AMELOGENESIS

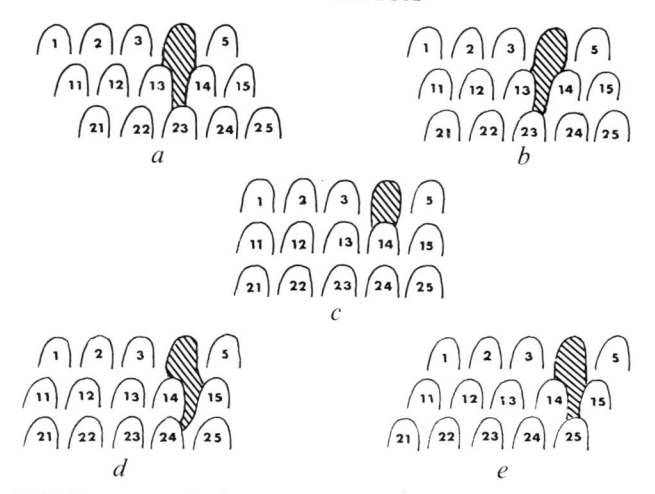

Fig. 15.10. Three rows of prisms are viewed end on at five different depths in the enamel. Note that as the rows cross each other an 'interprismatic region' appears when prisms are in line vertically (*c*). Such regions are commonly seen throughout human enamel and reinforce the suggestion that the 'keyhole' terminology is too awkward to be of much help in understanding enamel structure.

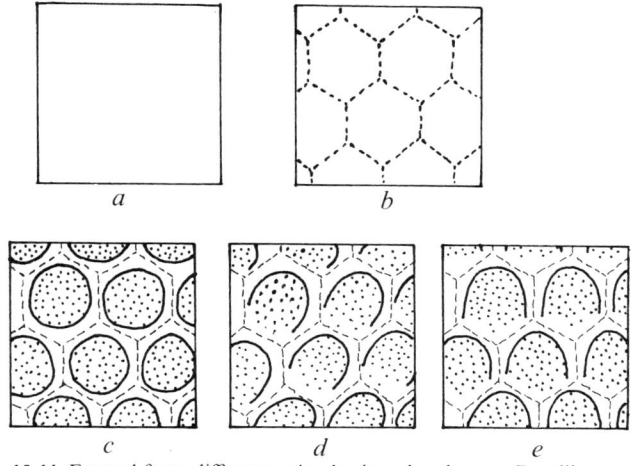

Fig. 15.11. Enamel from different animals viewed end on. *a*, Reptilian enamel (structureless). *b*, Mammal-like reptile with prisms but no interprismatic regions. *c*, *d*, and *e*, Different forms of recent mammalian enamel with prisms (stippled) and interprismatic regions. The relation between these and the ancestral enamel (*b*) is shown by the interrupted lines. (After Osborn and Hillman (1979) *Calc. Tiss. Res.* **29**, 47.)

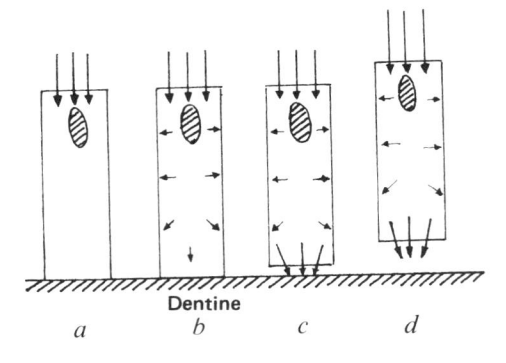

Fig. 15.12. A model used to account for the development of enamel and the movement of ameloblasts. For description, *see* text.

pressure to increase in the space initially enclosed between the mineralizing surface of the dentine and the united ends of the ameloblasts. When the pressure exceeds that at their basal ends, the ameloblasts are pushed backwards (*Fig. 15.12d*). This accounts for the origin of the force required to move ameloblasts and for the fact that the amount (length) of material secreted exactly matches the distance moved by the ameloblasts. The alternative, that ameloblast movement and secretion are independently controlled, seems very unlikely. However, Warshawsky (1978) suggested that the ameloblast is constantly growing in the region where the Tomes process joins the body of the ameloblast. This growth pushes the ameloblast away from the developing enamel. The growing Tomes process stays within the enamel where it is compressed by the growing prism and is 'literally forced out of existence'. Presumably the mineralizing prism grows (autonomously?) at the same rate as the ameloblast.

It can be visualized that material is flowing down the ameloblasts and that, as with flow along any tube, the material moves fastest down the centre and is almost stationary at the walls. This movement pushes out the originally flat ends of the cells into conical Tomes processes.

What might be the pattern of flow in the secreted material? This has been investigated in a smoke chamber (*Fig. 15.13*). The base of the smoke chamber is perforated by electrically heated screws, arranged in a hexagonal pattern. The chamber is covered with a glass roof. When the

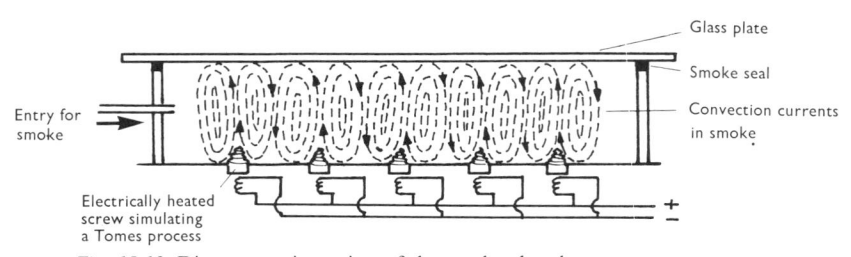

Fig. 15.13. Diagrammatic section of the smoke chamber.

screws are heated, convection currents from the hot points carry air to the glass roof where it is cooled and descends to the base. Smoke introduced to the chamber makes the convection currents visible: they are arranged in hexagonal 'cells', the centre being the upcurrent and the edges the downcurrent (*Fig. 15.14*). It is postulated that this is the pattern of flow in newly secreted enamel. There is an 'upcurrent' from the region in the middle of a Tomes process. Material is reflected back by the mineralizing enamel to produce a 'backcurrent' towards the edges of the Tomes processes. The enamel crystals lengthen within this current and are orientated parallel to the flow lines (*Fig. 15.15*). This orientation matches that on Face 1 in *Fig. 15.9*.

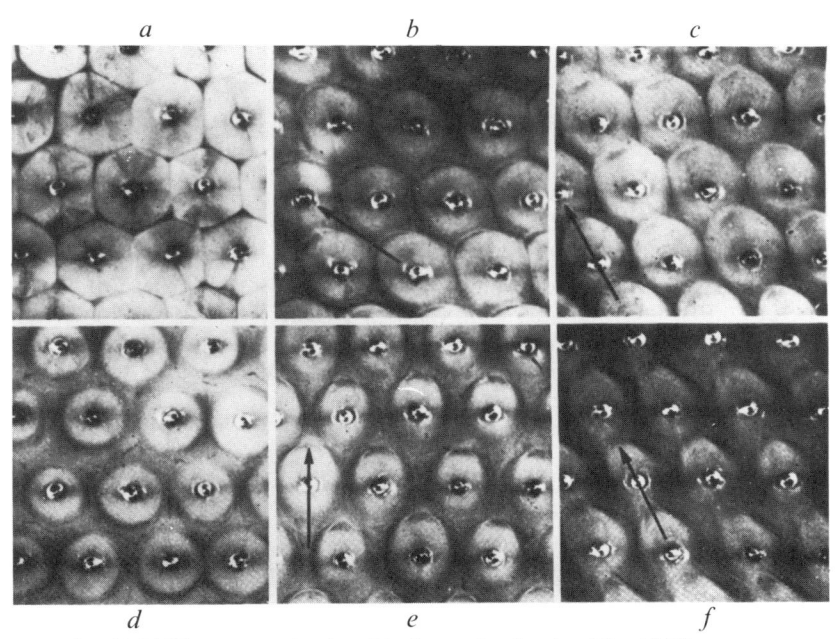

Fig. 15.14. The patterns developed in the smoke chamber (*Fig. 15.13*) are seen through its glass roof. Pattern *a* rapidly develops (cf. *Fig. 15.11b*) (screw tips can be seen in the centre of each 'convection cell'). Patterns *b* and *c* develop when Pattern *a* is distorted by pushing the glass roof over the convection cells in the directions shown by arrows (cf. *Figs. 15.11d* and *e*). After a few minutes Pattern *d* develops (cf. *Fig. 15.11c*). Pattern *e* and *f* are produced when Pattern *d* is sheaved. Similar shapes are also seen in the enamels of several mammals. (From Osborn J. W. (1970) *Calc. Tiss. Res.* **5**, 115.)

Early in amelogenesis the long axes of the ameloblasts become sharply angled to the direction in which they are moving when viewed in the longitudinal plane of the tooth (*Fig. 15.9*). The development of this angle is consistent with the hypothesis presented here and is described elsewhere

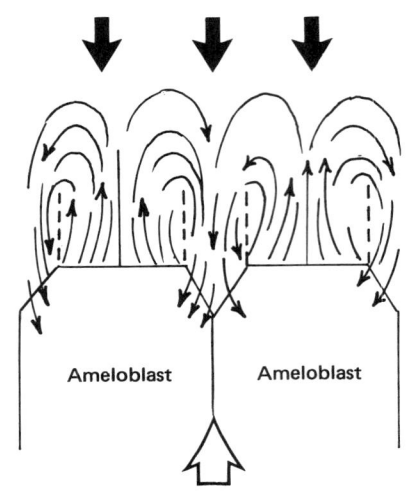

Fig. 15.15. If secreted material is 'reflected' by the mineralizing front, the smoke chamber (*Fig. 15.13*) predicts the above flow pattern in enamel matrix. The crystals are then orientated along the flow lines (cf. Face 1a in *Fig. 15.9*).

(Osborn, 1970*b*). The ameloblasts are now moving at an angle to the direction of the outflowing material. They are shearing the potentially hexagonal column of material they are secreting. (*Fig. 15.16*). The distortion of hexagons by shearing forces has been investigated in the smoke chamber and, according to the direction of shear, two of the three varieties of prism shape are produced—the horseshoe and the keyhole shapes (*Fig. 15.14*). It is worth mentioning that in the absence of shear the hexagonal patterns in the smoke chamber gradually become circular (*Fig. 15.14*), the other major variety of prism shape.

Returning to the Tomes processes it can readily be visualized that shear would distort them in the manner shown in *Fig. 15.9*. It can also be seen that little or no space is now available for secretion from their cuspal sides because these are now sliding past material which is flowing back (for absorption). Thus the cervical edge of the Tomes process undertakes the role of secretion and the cuspal edge that of absorption. The prism sheath develops at the border between outflow and backflow. The prism develops in the outflow and the interprismatic region in the backflow. Once again, crystals are orientated along the flow lines.

It can be seen that the 'prism region' in the smoke chamber merges 'cervically' into the 'interprismatic region' without a border line (*Fig. 15.14*). The border is only seen on the 'cuspal' side, as in human and most other enamels.

Finally, studies of the evolution of prisms in early mammals can be interpreted in support of the above hypothesis. They suggest that in reptiles there is no back flow during enamel formation because the crystals

AMELOGENESIS

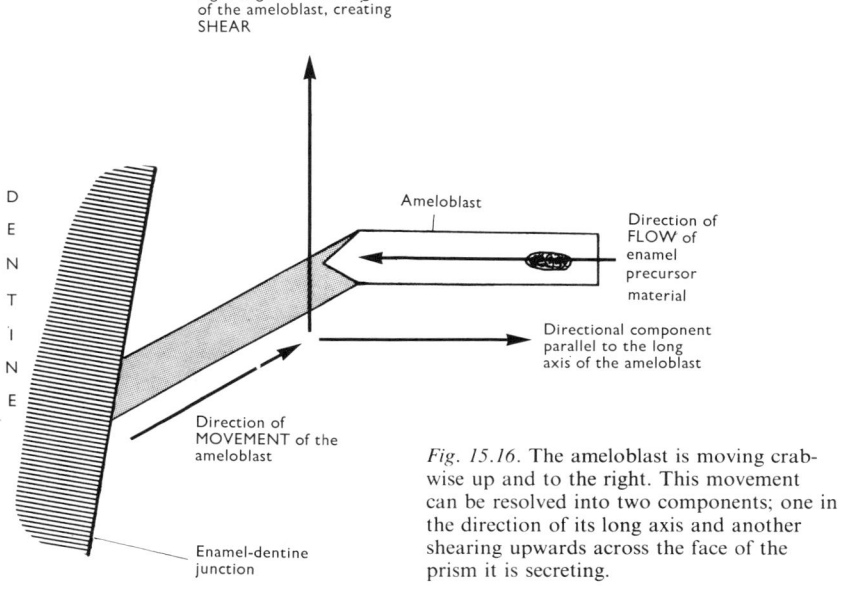

Fig. 15.16. The ameloblast is moving crabwise up and to the right. This movement can be resolved into two components; one in the direction of its long axis and another shearing upwards across the face of the prism it is secreting.

are parallel to each other and no prisms form (*Fig. 15.11a*). In early mammals hexagonal prisms are formed with no interprismatic region (*Fig. 15.11b*). This suggests there was backflow but no absorption. Lastly, both backflow and absorption led to the evolution of prisms separated by interprismatic regions (*Figs. 15.11c–e*) (cf. *figs. 15.14b–d*).

REFERENCES AND FURTHER READING

Burgess R. C. and Maclaren C. M. (1965) Proteins in developing bovine enamel. In: Stack M. V. and Fearnhead R. W. (ed.) *Tooth Enamel I*. Bristol, Wright.

Crabb H. S. M. and Darling A. I. (1962) *The Pattern of Progressive Mineralization in Human Dental Enamel*. Oxford, Pergamon.

Deporter D. A. and Ten Cate A. R. (1976) Fine structural localization of alkaline phosphatase in relation to enamel formation in the mouse molar. *Arch. Oral Biol.* **21**, 7.

Eastoe J. E. (1963) The amino-acid composition of proteins in dentine and enamel from developing human deciduous teeth. *Arch. Oral Biol.* **8**, 633.

Kallenbach E. (1968) Fine structure of rat incisor ameloblasts during enamel maturation. *J. Ultrastruct. Res.* **22**, 90.

Kallenbach E. (1977) Fine structure of the secretory ameloblasts of the kitten. *Am. J. Anat.* **148**, 479.

Nylen M. U., Eames E. D. and Omnell K. A. (1963) Crystal growth in rat enamel. *J. Cell Biol.* **18**, 109.

Osborn J. W. (1970a) The mechanism of prism formation in teeth: a hypothesis. *Calc. Tiss. Res.* **5**, 115.

Osborn J. W. (1970b) The mechanism of ameloblast movement: a hypothesis. *Calc. Tiss. Res.* **5**, 344.

Osborn J. W. (1974) Variations in structure and development of enamel. In: Melcher A. H. and Zarb G. A. (ed.), *Oral Sciences Reviews*, Vol. 3. Copenhagen, Munksgaard, p. 3.

Reith E. J. (1970) The stages of amelogenesis as observed in molar teeth of young rats. *J. Ultrastruct. Res.* **30**, 111.

Robinson C., Lowe N. R. and Weatherell J. A. (1977) Changes in amino-acid composition of developing rat incisor enamel. *Calc. Tiss. Res.* **23**, 19.

Ronnholm E. (1962a) The amelogenesis of human teeth as revealed by electron microscopy. II. The development of enamel crystallites. *J. Ultrastruct. Res.* **6**, 249.

Ronnholm E. (1962b) An electron microscopic study of amelogenesis in human teeth. I. The fine structure of ameloblasts. *J. Ultrastruct. Res.* **6**, 299.

Stack M. V. and Fearnhead H. W. (ed.) (1965) *Tooth Enamel I*. Bristol, Wright.

Warshawsky H. (1978) A freeze-fracture study of the topographic relationship between inner enamel–secretory ameloblasts in the rat incisor. *Am. J. Anat.* **152**, 153.

Young R. W. and Greulich R. C. (1963) Distinctive autoradiographic patterns of glycine incorporation in rat enamel and dentine matrices. *Arch. Oral Biol.* **8**, 509.

CHAPTER 16

ENAMEL STRUCTURE

To a light microscopist the unit of enamel is the prism. It seems probable that most prisms extend through the full thickness of the enamel, widening from a diameter of about 3 µm near the enamel–dentine junction to about 6 µm at the surface of the tooth. This widening is accounted for by the fact that near the enamel–dentine junction prisms are separated by larger interprismatic regions and also that the inner surface of the enamel has a smaller area than the outer surface. There is a little evidence that some prisms fail to reach the surface of the tooth from which it can be concluded that some ameloblasts might die before the full thickness of enamel is deposited.

PRISMS

Near the enamel–dentine junction, in true cross-section, human prisms may have any of the appearances shown in *Fig. 16.1a*. They are widely separated by an interprismatic region. At about 50 µm from the enamel–dentine junction they have enlarged considerably at the expense of the interprismatic region and are arranged as in *Fig. 16.1b*. At about 100 µm from the enamel–dentine junction they have the appearance shown in *Fig. 16.1c* and continue to appear like this until very close to the surface of the tooth, where they may again become very irregular (*Fig. 16.1d*) or their borders may disappear.

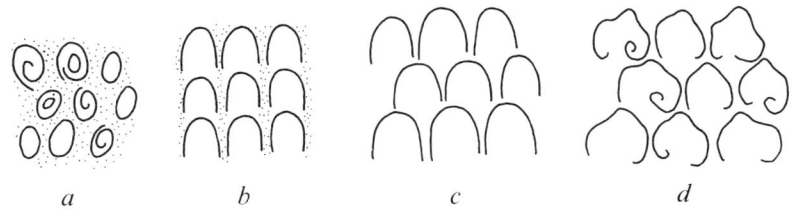

Fig. 16.1. Illustrating the appearances of human enamel prisms in cross-section: *a*, Close to the enamel–dentine junction; *b*, At about 50 µm from the enamel–dentine junction; *c*, Within most of the enamel; *d*, In some regions at the surface of the enamel. Generally agreed interprismatic regions are stippled.

Several texts still describe human enamel as consisting of 'keyhole-shaped' prisms (shaded in *Fig. 16.2b*), locked together in such a way that there is no interprismatic region. However, it is becoming increasingly popular to revert to the terminology which describes roughly circular prisms separated by an interprismatic region (*Fig. 16.2c*). Apart from a difference in crystal orientation, the latter region seems to be identical to that contained within the prism. It will be observed from the diagram that the two conflicting descriptions of human enamel structure (keyhole-shaped prisms without interprismatic regions and circular prisms separated by interprismatic regions) are related solely to differences in terminology. There is no disagreement about the structure being described (*Fig. 16.2a*). Both interpretations require the construction of imaginary lines in order to complete the prism border. Because there is general agreement that all other forms of prismatic enamel contain interprismatic regions it seems to us that it is less confusing, more consistent, and probably more realistic to describe human enamel prisms as roughly circular, bearing in mind that the prism body is in continuity with the interprismatic region cervically. A consideration of the relationship between ameloblasts and prisms suggests that the roughly circular shape approximates a 'tear-drop' (*see Fig. 15.9*) when prisms are not crossing each other.

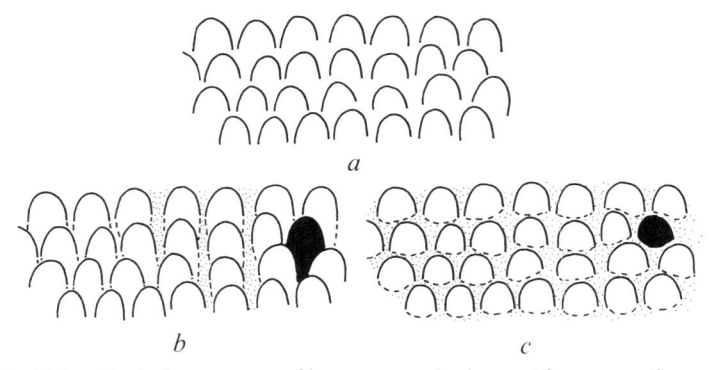

Fig. 16.2. a, Typical appearance of human enamel prisms cut in cross-section. One terminology refers to the majority of these prisms as being 'keyhole-shaped' (black prism in *b*) and recognizes interprismatic regions only where they are stippled in this diagram. The other terminology (*c*) refers to prisms as 'roughly circular' (black) and to the remaining region as being 'interprismatic'.

Prism Directions

In a longitudinally sectioned tooth (*Fig. 16.3a*) prisms seem to pass straight out approximately perpendicular to the enamel surface. In reality the prisms are bending from side to side (*Fig. 16.3b*) but these bends cannot be visualized in any one plane of section. The bends of each prism are slightly out of phase with those of vertically adjacent prisms (*Fig. 16.3c*). It can be seen that when a block of such prisms (*Fig. 16.3d*) is cut,

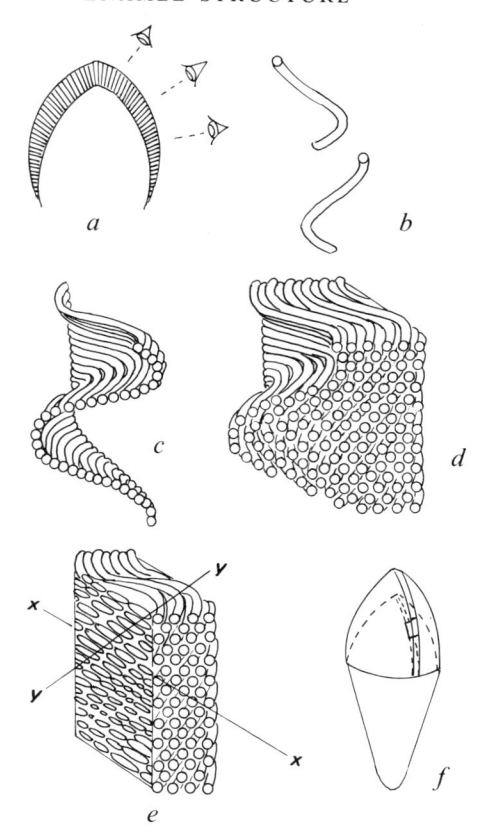

Fig. 16.3. When viewed end on (*a*) prisms bend from side to side as they pass to the surface (*b*). Each prism starts out from the enamel–dentine junction in a slightly different direction from its vertically adjacent neighbours (*c*). Laterally adjacent prisms are roughly parallel to each other (*d*). When a block such as *d* is longitudinally sectioned the cut face contains sectioned profiles of prisms (*e*) but because the cervical sides of prisms are invisible the cut surface usually appears to contain uninterrupted prisms passing through the full thickness of the enamel in the direction *x–x*. Bands of parazones and diazones pass in the direction *y–y* which is roughly equivalent to the direction of the Hunter–Schreger bands.

the sectioned surface should contain lines of sectioned profiles (*Fig. 16.3e*) instead of the apparently straight prisms which are normally seen (*Fig. 16.3a*). However, these sectioned profiles can generally only be seen if the surface of the ground section is etched with acid and then stained. In such a section oblique rows of more longitudinally sectioned prisms are separated by rows of more transversely sectioned prisms (left face of *Fig.*

16.3e), the so-called parazone–diazone appearance. The rows pass upwards and outwards at an angle to the enamel surface. It is sufficient to state, without explanation, the existence and directions of the obliquely orientated rows of parazones and diazones are entirely consistent with the remainder of *Fig. 16.3*. These oblique rows represent one of several ways in which the Hunter–Schreger bands (*see later*) can be visualized.

Each apparently longitudinally sectioned prism in *Fig. 16.3a* actually consists of a string of obliquely sectioned prisms (*x–x* in *Fig. 16.3e*) whose sides are invisible unless the surface is etched and stained.

When a longitudinal section of a tooth is viewed by *reflected* light the enamel is crossed by oblique light and dark bands, parallel to the (usually invisible) parazones and diazones, which curve cuspally and outwards from the enamel–dentine junction about three quarters of the way to the surface. These are the Hunter–Schreger bands (*Fig. 16.4*). If the light source is moved from the left side of the microscope (for example) to the right side, the light and dark bands become reversed. The effect is an epiphenomenon due to the fact that the sides of prisms (or the crystals of which they are composed) reflect light.

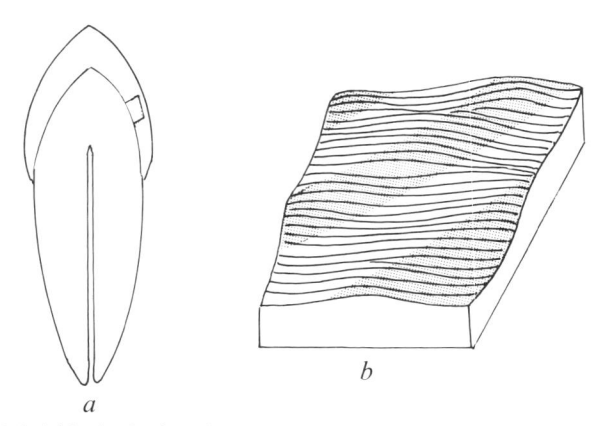

Fig. 16.4. A block of prisms has been removed from the position shown in *a*. Within the thickness of the block prisms bend from side to side (*b*) producing the Hunter-Schreger bands (which pass outwards and upwards).

As a first approximation it is helpful to think of human enamel as consisting of a series of single-prism thick, coaxial, hollow cones with open apices lying against the enamel–dentine junction and their free edges at the surface of the tooth (*Fig. 16.5*). Each cone is a single layer of undulating tapered prisms. The phase difference between the bends of prisms contained in adjacent cones has been described above. At the tip of the cusp the apical angles of the cones are so acute that most longitudinal sections of a tooth cut the faces of several cones and the phase differences

ENAMEL STRUCTURE

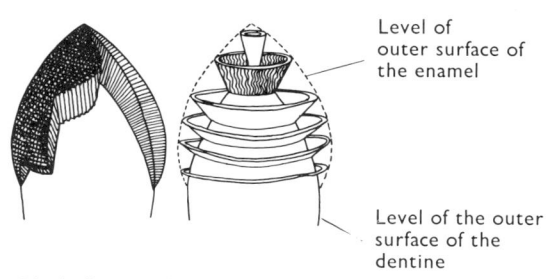

Fig. 16.5. Block diagrams illustrating the structure of enamel.

between the undulating prisms contained in each of the cones are superimposed on each other. The resultant apparent intertwining of prisms produces a gnarled appearance (gnarled enamel) which obscures a regularity of structure which can only be observed in transverse sections of the tooth taken through the cuspal enamel.

Contrary to previous descriptions, prisms in the cervical region of permanent teeth are not directed outwards and cervically but are generally approximately horizontal.

Cross Striations

When viewed in the light microscope prisms are often crossed by narrow bands about 4 µm apart known as cross-striations (*Fig. 16.6a*). Scanning electron micrographs appear to show that prisms may be alternately varicose and constricted (*Fig. 16.6c*), adjacent varicosities being separated by about 4 µm. Reconstructions of enamel prisms (*Fig. 16.7*) suggest that prisms undulate with a periodicity of about 4 µm (*Fig. 16.6b*). It may be noted that if the former interpretation were correct adjacent cross-striations would be expected to be staggered. But they are in line. Finally, sections of an undulating prism produce an alternately varicose and constricted outline (*Fig. 16.6d*).

It has been suggested, without evidence, that the cross-striations may be related to regular variations in the organic/inorganic ratio of substances or to variations in crystal size. Whatever their optical basis, the cross-striations are thought to represent daily increments of prism growth.

Prism Sheath

To the light microscopist the prism sheath appears to be about 0·5 µm wide but electron microscopy reveals that it is at most about 0·1 µm wide. A rapidly diminishing number of electron microscopists consider that a sheath *per se* does not exist and that a prism is bounded solely by an interface between crystallites of different orientation. However, a close

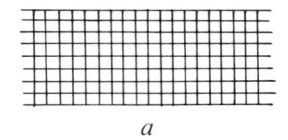

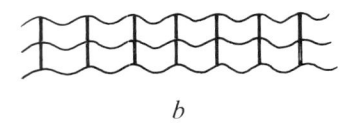

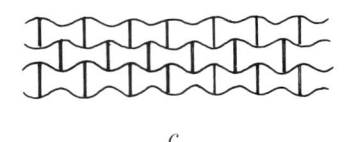

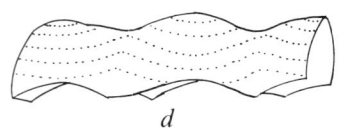

Fig. 16.6. Cross-striations are about 4 μm apart (*a*), approximately equal to the widths of prisms. One view is that cross-striations correspond to undulations of prisms (*b*), another that they correspond to varicosities and constrictions (*c*). However, the latter view seems to imply that cross-striations would be out of phase, which they are not. Note that if an undulating prism were sectioned horizontally (*d*) the cut surface would appear varicose and constricted.

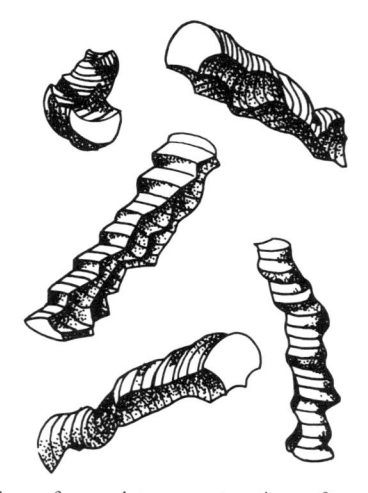

Fig. 16.7. Drawings of wax-plate reconstructions of enamel prisms.

study of electron micrographs which have been considered to demonstrate this interface seems always to reveal an irregular crystallite-free region (a region of microporosity) where the cervical ends of the crystallites in the more cuspal prism unevenly abut against the sides of the crystallites in the cervically adjacent prism (*Fig. 16.8*).

ENAMEL STRUCTURE

Fig. 16.8. Typical appearance of the border between two longitudinally sectioned prisms. There is a region of microporosity between the cervical border of the more cuspal prism and the cuspal border of the more cervical prism.

It is necessary to explain how a prism sheath, 0·1 μm wide, can be seen. Under ideal conditions the light microscope only has a resolving power of about 0·2 μm. In spite of this, sheaths can be seen even at low magnifications.

A plausible explanation has been based on measurements of interference fringes seen in light micrographs (Osborn and Roberts, 1970). Their observations suggest there is a sudden change in refractive index between the protein sheath (R.I. $\simeq$ 1·3) and the crystals of the prism (R.I. $\simeq$ 1·7). Light is totally internally reflected at this boundary if it strikes the border at grazing angles less than 35°. The failure of light to pass through the boundary leads to a huge increase in the apparent width of the sheaths (*Fig. 16.9*).

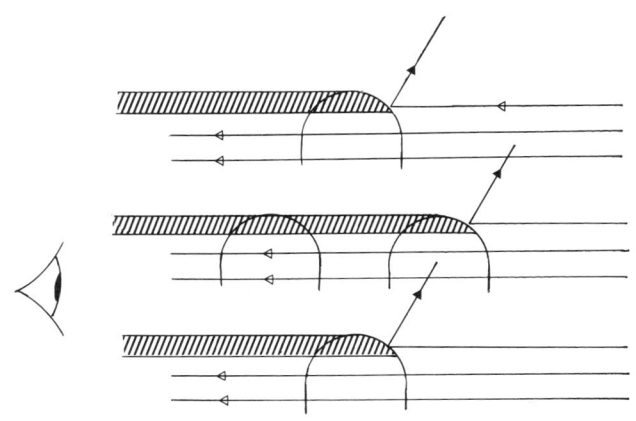

Fig. 16.9. The sides of prisms passing vertically out of the page are viewed by transmitted light passing from the right. Light is reflected where it grazes the sheath and this produces the appearance of a sheath far thicker than it really is.

Within approximately 12 μm of the surface of the enamel, in many regions the crystallites are all parallel to the long axes of the prisms and the irregular, microporous, crystallite-free prism sheath no longer exists.

The enamel in these regions therefore appears structureless to the light microscopist. The parallel arrangement (and therefore closer packing) of the crystallites and the absence of prism sheaths probably accounts for the observation that the surface enamel is the most highly mineralized.

The enamel surface of recently erupted and unerupted teeth has been studied by scanning electron microscopy. Although the majority of deciduous teeth contain regions in which the surface is structureless, such regions are far less common in permanent teeth. The perikymata (*see below*) crests may be structureless but prism outlines are nearly always visible in the troughs. These outlines often surround depressions about 2 μm deep which were, presumably, once occupied by the ageing ameloblasts. In some regions small hollow hillocks of enamel up to 50 μm wide may project from the surface. The tops of these hillocks may be broken off to reveal irregular craters.

ENAMEL POROSITY

When sections of enamel are placed in aqueous solutions of certain substances some of the solution diffuses into the enamel and changes its optical properties, particularly the degree of birefringence. The change in birefringence can be measured and is related to the refractive index of the aqueous solution and the amount that diffuses into the enamel. Since the refractive index of the solution is known the amount that has diffused into the enamel can be calculated. It is found that the size of the molecules of the dissolved substance determines the amount which can penetrate into the spaces in the enamel and it is assumed that the volume diffusing when the solution of smallest molecular size is used represents the volume of spaces present in enamel. In this way it can be shown that enamel contains a system of micropores which act as a molecular sieve and that the volume of pores is about 0–2 per cent of the enamel volume. Attempts have been made to show that the optical properties of the striae of Retzius (*see below*) and the cross-striations are related to differences in the amounts of pores present in them as compared with the rest of the enamel.

BROWN STRIAE AND PERIKYMATA

The brown striae of Retzius seem to reflect a further phasic nature of enamel formation. The cross-striations are probably related to daily increments whereas the striae appear to be 4-day to 16-day increments.

It is generally supposed that, like the cross-striations, the striae are formed in relation to some systemic influence. Two features support this contention. First, neonatal lines seem to be well-marked striae. Second, it has sometimes been observed that, taking into account the times at which they have been formed, the striae in all the teeth of a dentition are the same. In other words, the supposed systemic stimulus affected all developing teeth at the same time. However, so far the evidence for this latter conclusion seems limited. In many sections of enamel, striae are invisible because they are oblique to the plane of section; they can usually be seen if the section is tilted under the microscope.

It is a simple enough matter to observe brown striae but it has been found very difficult to give a uniform description of them. They may be between 150 μm thick down to the thickness of a cross-striation, they may be hypo- or hypermineralized, they may be continuous or discontinuous, and clear striae, as opposed to brown, have also been described. The borders of prisms within the thicker brown striae are particularly optically dense and it may be that the brown colour is due to blue light (short wavelength) being abnormally scattered at these borders. This is supported by the observation that striae are blue-white when seen by reflected light. It has been speculated without evidence that within striae crystallites may be larger or smaller and that they may be orientated differently from crystallites in adjacent regions (similar speculations have been made on enamel structure in the region of the cross-striations).

It has been reported that in association with striae prisms may bend cervically or that they may bend in the transverse plane of the tooth.

If this latter observation is true, prisms have three 'curvatures'. A primary curvature (cf. dentinal tubules) is responsible for the Hunter–Schreger band appearance and has a periodicity of about 1000 μm. A secondary curvature with a periodicity which may be from about 100 μm to about 16 μm is related to the striae of Retzius. A tertiary curvature, or undulation, with a periodicity of 4 μm is related to the cross-striations (*Fig. 16.10*).

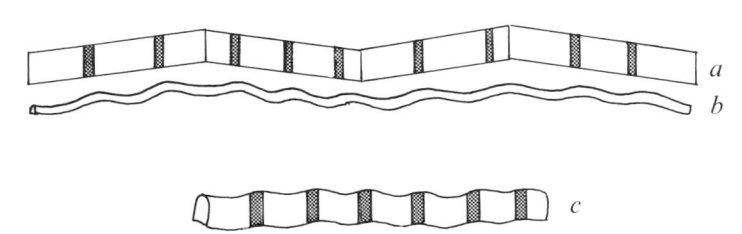

Fig. 16.10. Prisms bend from side to side to produce the Hunter–Schreger bands (*a*). A further shorter periodicity of undulation may be associated with the striae of Retzius (*b*). A still shorter periodicity may correspond with the cross-striations (*c*).

A series of fine furrows and ridges surround the surface of young teeth. These are called 'perikymata' (*peri* = around, *kyma* = wave). Ground longitudinal sections of teeth show that the brown striae meet the enamel surface at the furrows. This suggests the following (*Fig. 16.11*). At fairly regular time intervals all secreting ameloblasts may be temporarily

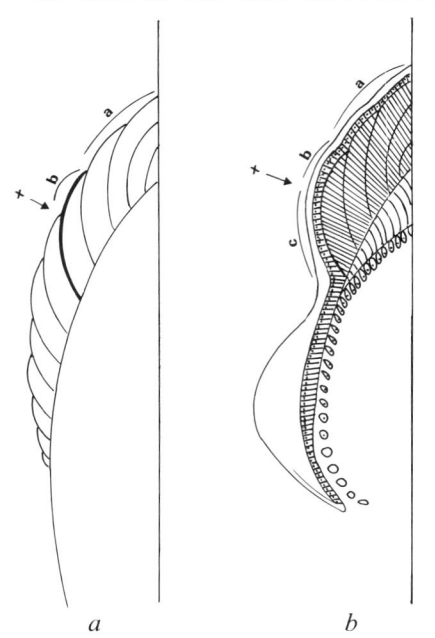

Fig. 16.11. Perikymata in the finished tooth are shown in *a*. Their development is visualized in *b*. Ameloblasts *a* have completed their secretory cycle. Ameloblasts *b* and *c* are secreting prisms. At a later stage ameloblasts *b* and *c* stop secreting but *c* start up again a little later. A furrow, *x*, is developed on the tooth surface between the prisms secreted by ameloblasts *b* and *c*.

affected in some way and a stria is formed. Most of them return to normal activity. But the oldest of these ameloblasts do not recover and become solely absorptive. The junction between these now absorptive ameloblasts and the 'rejuvenated' ameloblasts is represented by a furrow on the enamel surface.

Although pits, which were once occupied by the Tomes processes, can be recognized over much of the surface of a newly erupted tooth, they cannot usually be distinguished in the furrows of the perikymata. All developmental surface irregularities tend to be obliterated by abrasion after the tooth has erupted leaving a flat surface scored by scratches. This is generally covered by cuticle or plaque and, occasionally, small islands of (ectopic) cement.

LAMELLAE, TUFTS AND SPINDLES

Three further features of enamel can be seen in ground sections. Enamel lamellae are irregular vertical sheets of organic or hypomineralized matrix

ENAMEL STRUCTURE

extending from the tooth surface often as far as, and occasionally beyond, the enamel–dentine junction (*Fig. 16.12*). It has been suggested that they develop along planes of tension within the developing enamel, a slight disturbance leading to a failure of mineralization along the plane. Second, some of these lamellae may open up during development and cells from the enamel organ collect in the cleft. Finally, with advancing age, a third type of lamella may form in which the underlying dentine tends to contract so that the enamel, now unsupported, fractures. Organic material from the oral cavity then collect in the split.

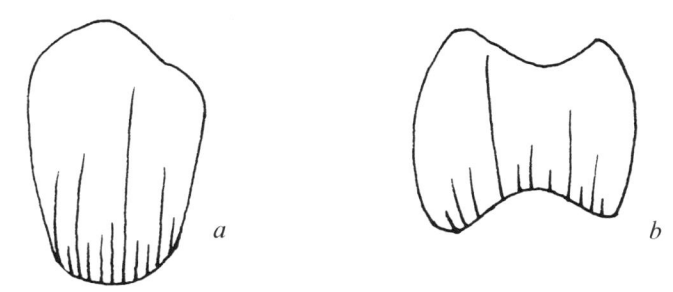

Fig. 16.12. The crown of an extracted tooth is submerged in acid for an hour. It is then washed and stained with haemotoxylin. The stain is picked up by lamellae. The distribution of lamellae in a canine (*a*) and premolar (*b*) are shown.

Groups of ribbon-like structures extend from the enamel–dentine junction into the enamel for up to one-third of its thickness. These constitute the 'enamel tufts', so called on account of their resemblance, when seen in transverse ground sections of teeth, to tufts of grass. A reconstruction of a small part of a tuft is shown in *Fig. 16.13*. Each tuft consists of a number of disconnected 'leaves' which appear to coincide with thickenings of the prism sheaths. In a recent study it was pointed out that when a substance changes from the liquid to the solid state contractions occur. In enamel, hydroxyapatite changes from the ionic (liquid) state in the ameloblast secretions to the solid state in the enamel crystallites. With the change of state, contractions will be expected and it is possible that these contractions could lead to the widening of prism sheaths which corresponds with the tufts. Evidently the tufts will follow the direction of prisms.

It was suggested in Chapter 12 that odontoblasts produce a greater length of process than the distance they move. At the start of dentinogenesis processes are pushed between pre-ameloblasts, particularly in the cuspal region. Subsequently, enamel develops around these processes leaving 'enamel tubules'. In human enamel these are very short and

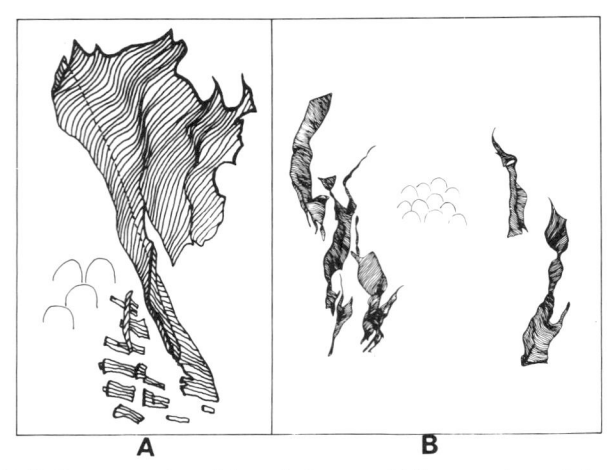

Fig. 16.13. Reconstruction of the tufts in enamel. The enamel cusp is towards the top and the cervical margin towards the bottom. The prism outlines included in each reconstruction are about 5 µm wide.

known as enamel spindles. The spindles lie parallel to the long axes of the pre-ameloblasts (not the prisms) and probably become mineralized.

REFERENCES AND FURTHER READING

Boyde A. (1969) Electron microscopic observations relating to the nature and development of prism decussation in mammalian dental enamel. *Bull Group Int. Rech. Sci. Stomatol. Odontol.* **12**, 151.

Fosse G. (1964) The number of prism bases on the inner and outer surface of the enamel mantle of human teeth. *J. Dent. Res.* **43**, 57.

Fosse G. (1968) A quantitative analysis of the numerical density and the distributional pattern of prisms and ameloblasts in dental enamel and tooth germs. *Acta Odont. Scand.* **26**, 573.

Fujita T. (1939) Über die Retzius'schen Parallelstreifen des Zahnschmelzes. *Anat. Anz.* **86**, 350.

Glas J. E. and Nylen M. U. (1965) A correlated electron microscopical and microradiographic study of human enamel. *Arch. Oral Biol* **10**, 893.

Gustafson A. (1959) A morphologic investigation of certain variations in the structure and mineralization of human dental enamel. *Odont. Tidskr.* **67**, 361.

Gustafson G. and Gustafson A. (1967) Microanatomy and histochemistry of enamel. In: Miles A. E. W. (ed.), *Structural and Chemical Organization of Teeth*, vol. 2. New York, Academic.

Gustafson F. and Silness J. (1969) Crystal shape in the prism sheath region of sound human enamel. *Acta Odont. Scand.* **27**, 617.

Helmcke J.-G. (1967) Ultrastructure of enamel. In: Miles A. E. W. (ed.), *Structural and Chemical Organization of Teeth,* vol. 2. New York, Academic.

Heuser H. (1961) Die Struktur des menslichen Zahnschmelzes in Oberflach in histogischen Bild (replica Technik). *Arch. Oral Biol.* **4**, 50.
Johnson N. W. (1967) Some aspects of the ultrastructure of early human enamel caries seen with the electron microscope. *Arch. Oral Biol.* **12**, 1505.
Meckel A. H., Griebstein W. J. and Neal R. J. (1965) Structure of mature human dental enamel as observed by electron microscopy. *Arch. Oral Biol.* **10**, 775.
Osborn J. W. (1965) The nature of the Hunter–Schreger bands in enamel. *Arch. Oral Biol.* **10**, 929.
Osborn J. W. (1968a) Directions and inter-relationships of enamel prisms from the sides of human teeth. *J. Dent. Res.* **47**, 223.
Osborn J. W. (1968b) Directions and inter-relationships of prisms in cuspal and cervical enamel of human teeth. *J. Dent. Res.* **47**, 395.
Osborn J. W. (1969) The three-dimensional morphology of the tufts in human enamel. *Acta Anat.* **73**, 481.
Osborn J. W. (1974) Variations in the structure and development of enamel. In: Melcher A. H. and Zarb G. A. (ed.), *Oral Sciences Reviews*, vol. 3. Copenhagen, Munksgaard, p. 3.
Osborn J. W. and Roberts A. M. (1970) Optical fringe effects of prism borders in human enamel. *J. Microsc.* **93**, 123.
Poole D. F. G. and Brooks A. W. (1961) The arrangement of crystallites in enamel prisms. *Arch. Oral Biol.* **5**, 14.
Ripa L. W., Gwinnett A. J. and Buonocoré M. G. (1965) The prismless outer layer of deciduous and permanent enamel. In: Melcher A. H. and Zarb G. A. (ed.), *Oral Sciences Reviews*, vol. 5. Copenhagen, Munksgaard, p. 41.
Schour I. and Hoffman M. M. (1939) Studies in tooth development. II. The rate of apposition of enamel and dentine in man and other mammals. *J. Dent. Res.* **18**, 161.
Stack M. V. and Fearnhead R. W. (ed.) (1965) *Tooth Enamel.* Bristol, Wright.
Whittaker D. K. and Richards D. (1978) Scanning electron microscopy of the neonatal line in human enamel. *Arch. Oral Biol.* **23**, 45.

CHAPTER 17

CEMENTOGENESIS AND CEMENT STRUCTURE

INTRODUCTION

Cementogenesis intermittently continues, usually at a very slow pace, throughout life. Like all mineralized tissues a matrix is secreted and subsequently mineralized and, like dentine, there is usually an unmineralized layer, precement (= cementoid), on its surface.

Cement (= cementum) is classified in three ways. *Primary cement* is the first-formed cement which covers about the coronal two-thirds of the root. It is followed by *secondary cement* which covers the apical two-thirds of the root including the associated primary cement. Cement may or may not contain cementocytes lying in lacunae. This feature leads to a second classification. Primary cement is nearly always acellular. This *acellular cement* is followed by *cellular cement*. In the same way that it is often difficult to distinguish between primary and secondary dentine, so it is often difficult to distinguish between primary and secondary cement unless one uses the criterion, presence (or absence) of lacunae. However, acellular cement often covers or mingles with cellular cement so that the equivalence between primary and acellular cement breaks down.

The last classification of cement, and the one used here, is based on the origin of its matrix fibres. The matrix may contain intrinsic fibres derived from cementoblasts or extrinsic fibres derived from the periodontal ligament. The latter are the Sharpey fibres of cement. The classification recognizes *extrinsic, mixed* and *intrinsic fibre cements*. In addition, all three classifications would add *afibrillar cement* and *intermediate cement*.

AFIBRILLAR 'CEMENT' OR HYALINE 'DENTINE'?

The apical region of a developing root is covered by a growing intact Hertwig's root sheath. Adjacent to and inside the sheath odontoblasts differentiate. They send out small processes towards the basal lamina separating them from the sheath and then move back while depositing the first dentine matrix. The inner portion of this early matrix is now mineralized leaving an outer unmineralized layer about 1 μm or more thick (Owens, 1976, 1980). At the same time the epithelial cells of the root sheath (which contain some rough endoplasmic reticulum) secrete material which mixes with this unmineralized dentine matrix, and the basal lamina breaks up (*see Fig. 12.2*). The root sheath now fragments and the epithelial cells migrate away from the root surface while cells of the dental follicle migrate towards the root surface. These ectomesenchymal cells from the investing layer of the follicle differentiate and develop several processes directed towards the unmineralized, hybrid, root surface tissue and initiate its mineralization.

The hybrid tissue covering the dentine may contain so few collagen fibres in the cervical region of the tooth as to be termed *afibrillar cement* (despite the fact that very little of its matrix comes from the newly differentiated cementoblasts). This thin strip of tissue lying along the whole root is more highly mineralized than the adjacent dentine and is probably the same tissue as that known as the hyaline layer of dentine. It is noteworthy that no matrix vesicles have been demonstrated in association with the mineralization of cement.

Much of the following analysis of cementogenesis is based on the descriptions of Jones (1981).

EXTRINSIC FIBRE CEMENT

The cementoblasts covering the afibrillar cement are oval cells with their long axes parallel to the root surface towards which they send short cell processes. They contain only modest amounts of rough endoplasmic reticulum, Golgi apparatus and secretory vesicles. With the migration of the root sheath cells away from the root surface, collagen fibres of the dental follicle come to lie against the mineralizing afibrillar cement and between the newly differentiated cementoblasts (*Fig. 17.1*). The cementoblasts secrete mainly non-fibrillar components into and around these

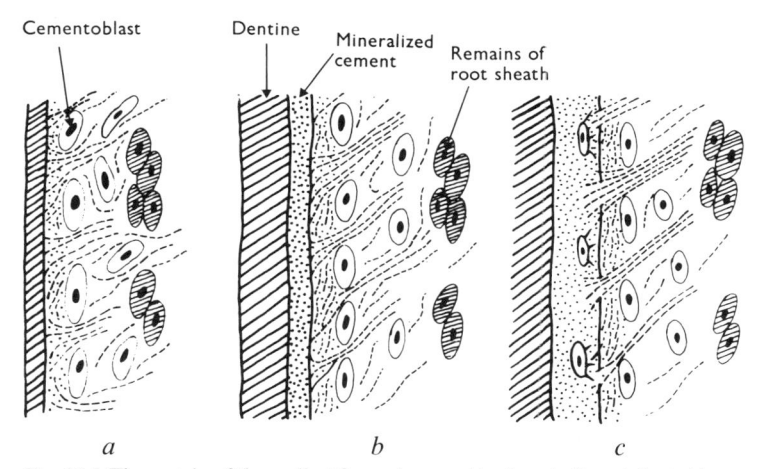

Fig. 17.1. The matrix of the earliest formed cement is almost all contributed by the periodontal ligament rather than by cementoblasts (*a*). In later formed cement (*b*) and (*c*) progessively more matrix may be secreted by cementoblasts. The cores of the Sharpey fibres may not mineralize (*c*).

extrinsic collagen fibres, together comprising precement, and organize their mineralization to become *extrinsic fibre cement*. In this situation extrinsic fibre cement is synonymous with primary cement and (the first-formed) acellular cement.

The collagen of the extrinsic fibres is grouped into thick bundles (Sharpey fibres) about 6 μm wide whose cores mineralize more rapidly than their peripheries. In SEM photomicrographs the surface of the cement may therefore be covered by tightly packed shallow domes, each dome being the mineralizing projection of a bundle of collagen fibres. Note that the fibrous matrix of this cement is produced by fibroblasts in the dental follicle.

MIXED FIBRE CEMENT

Extrinsic fibre cement develops while the tooth is erupting. It is generally followed by the development of mixed fibre cement around the apical two-thirds of the root. The 'mixed' refers to a matrix which is composed of extrinsic fibres from the ligament and intrinsic fibres produced by cementoblasts. The extrinsic fibres, as before, are arranged roughly perpendicular to the tooth surface and are the Sharpey fibres whose extensions across the ligament are buried in the alveolar bone. The intrinsic fibres are roughly parallel to the root surface and weave a lattice around the extrinsic fibres similar to the matrix of circumpulpal dentine. The intrinsic fibres mineralize more rapidly than the extrinsic fibres and from them mineralization spreads into the periphery of the extrinsic fibres. The surface of a dried tooth covered by mixed fibre cement is therefore pitted by hollows which at one time contained the unmineralized cores of Sharpey fibres (cf. the opposite, domed, appearance of extrinsic fibre cement).

INTRINSIC FIBRE CEMENT

This contains no extrinsic fibres and, therefore, no Sharpey fibres. Clearly it does not support the tooth in the socket. The fibres are parallel to the root surface and grouped into irregular regions containing fibres parallel to each other in the plane of the surface. The mineralization front is parallel to the root surface which therefore appears flat; no extrinsic fibres exist to distort the shape of the mineralizing front.

SIGNIFICANCE OF FIBRE FORMS

The type of fibre cement formed seems to depend on the rate of its formation. The first-formed, extrinsic fibre, cement develops while the tooth is erupting to reach the occlusal plane. It is a thin layer, not rapidly formed. When the tooth has reached the occlusal plane the root grows backwards into the jaws, the intrusive phase of root development, and a rather more rapidly formed thicker layer of mixed fibre cement is developed over the apical two-thirds of the root. Both of the first-formed cements are capable of suspending the tooth in its socket due to the incorporation of extrinsic fibres.

Through life the movements of the tooth, as its position is adjusted to compensate for wear, lead to narrowing or widening the periodontal ligament according to the direction of movement. It appears that for optimum function the width of the ligament is critical and, in compensation for the movement, either bone is resorbed to widen it or cement is deposited to narrow it. The type of cement deposited seems related to the speed at which compensation is required. Slow movement results in extrinsic fibre cement which includes few or no cementocytes; rapid movement, such as that following the extraction of adjacent teeth, results in intrinsic fibre cement which contains many cementocytes and functions to correct the width of the ligament rather than to support the tooth; an intermediate rate of movement results in mixed fibre cement which may or may not include cementocytes.

INTERMEDIATE CEMENT

On the surface of the root dentine in premolars and molars a variety of cement characterized by wide irregular branching spaces is frequently found. This is the intermediate cement. The origin of the cells that at one time occupied these spaces is in dispute. It has been suggested that these spaces once contained epithelial cells derived from Hertwig's root sheath that had become trapped on the dentine surface during the formation of the first layers of dentine. Evidence for this is based on studies of rodents. An alternative is that during eruption of the cheek teeth cementocytes, whose processes have become attached to the cement and whose periodontal surface is attached to the connective tissue, become pulled upwards and distorted by movement of the erupting tooth. A study of dogs indicates that the lacunae in this type of cement are occupied by odontoblasts which are trapped on the outer surface of the dentine at the start of dentinogenesis, subsequently being engulfed by the forming cement. The different interpretations of intermediate cement are the result of species differences.

CEMENT STRUCTURE

In purely descriptive terms cement may be cellular or acellular. Cellular cement contains cementocytes trapped in lacunae. The further the cementocytes are from the surface of the cement the fewer the organelles they contain and the smaller they become. Far from the surface they may be dead and leave empty lacunae. Cementocytes have cell processes which extend into canaliculi largely radiating outwards from the lacunae towards the periodontal ligament, their source of nutrition. Towards the surface the cementocytes maintain contact with the adjacent cementoblasts by means of these cell processes through the medium of gap and tight junctions. Presumably the functional significance of this arrangement is the maintenance of a nutritive pathway which is not totally dependent on simple diffusion through canaliculi. It is not easy to understand the value of maintaining live cementocytes in the lacunae unless the cells have some function in supporting the mineralized matrix (including Sharpey fibres) which entombs them.

Cement, in one of its several forms, covers the anatomical root of the tooth. It is said that in 60 per cent of cases it overlaps the enamel, in 30 per cent of cases it meets the enamel edge to edge, and in 10 per cent of cases there is a gap between enamel and dentine. Clearly these figures relate to newly erupted teeth since in old age where much of the anatomical root has been exposed the cement has frequently been worn away to expose the dentine. Closer examination of tooth surfaces by scanning electron microscopy commonly reveals microscopic islands of cement patchily distributed over the cervical enamel. Whether they are afibrillar or fibre cement, and whether they have any clinical significance are not known.

Cement is deposited over the apex of the tooth and is the prime reason for the narrowing of the apical canal with age.

Cement contains incremental lines whose separation depends on the rate of cement formation. Therefore they tend to be closest together in extrinsic (usually acellular) fibre cement. Because it is more heavily mineralized than intrinsic (usually cellular) fibre cement, the radio-dense incremental lines are less obvious in extrinsic fibre cement.

When cement thickness is plotted against age for a large number of individuals it can be seen that its thickness increases with age. Cement thickness is one of the criteria used in forensic medicine to estimate the age of an individual from whom a tooth has been recovered.

Cement is readily resorbed during the shedding of deciduous teeth. Evidence of cement resorption is commonly seen towards the apices of permanent teeth. Patches of cement are removed by osteoclasts and the area subsequently repaired by the formation of new cement thereby leaving a reversal line in the mineralized tissue.

Spurs of the cement sometimes project into the periodontal ligament. Presumably these are largely extrinsic fibre cement, mineralization having spread outwards along adjacent Sharpey fibres. Occasionally irregular cement-like bodies are seen free within the ligament. These *cementicles* may later become attached to the tooth as cement spreads into the ligament. Abnormal thickening of cement is referred to as *hyper-*

cementosis. Provided the area of hypercementosis contains extrinsic fibres the region attaches the tooth more firmly by increasing the area of attachment. If it is a pure intrinsic fibre cement its only function would be to maintain an optimum periodontal thickness.

When a functioning tooth moves through the alveolar bone, the bone rather than the cement is nearly always resorbed. It has sometimes been argued that the tooth is protected by precement (= cementoid). Perhaps this is a semantic problem because a region covered by precement indicates an area of cement formation and could hardly be simultaneously an area of resorption.

REFERENCES AND FURTHER READING

Bernard G. W. (1970) Initial calcification of cementum. Abstract of a paper given at the 48th meeting of the International Association for Dental Research. *J. Dent. Res.* Supplement.

Boyde A. and Jones S. J. (1972) Scanning electron microscope studies of the formation of mineralized tissues. In: Slavkin H. C. and Bavetta L. A. (ed.), *Developmental Aspects of Oral Biology.* London, Academic, p. 243.

Furseth R. (1969) The fine structure of the cellular cementum of young human teeth. *Arch. Oral Biol.* **14**, 1147.

Jones S. J. (1981) Cement. In: Osborn J. W. (ed.), *Dental Anatomy and Embryology.* Oxford, Blackwell.

Lester K. (1969) The incorporation of epithelial cells by cementum. *J. Ultrastruct. Res.* **27**, 63.

Listgartern M. A. (1970) Ultrastructure of cementogenesis in human teeth. Abstract of a paper given at the 48th meeting of the International Association for Dental Research. *J. Dent. Res.* Supplement.

Owens P. D. A. (1972) Light microscope observations on the formation of the layer of Hopewell-Smith in human teeth. *Arch. Oral Biol.* **17**, 1985.

Owens P. D. A. (1974) A light microscopic study of the development of the roots of premolar teeth in dogs. *Arch. Oral Biol.* **20**, 709.

Owens P. D. A. (1976) The root surface in human teeth: a microradiographic study. *J. Anat.* **122**, 389.

Owens P. D. A. (1980) A light and electron microscopic study of the early stages of root surface formation in molar teeth in the rat. *Arch Oral Biol.* **24**, 901.

Selvig K. A. (1964) Ultrastructural study of cementum formation. *Acta Odont. Scand.* **22**, 105.

CHAPTER 18

ROOT FORMATION

It will be recalled from reading Chapter 3 that the outer and inner enamel epithelia are continuous at the cervical edge of the dental organ, forming the cervical loop. In the late bell stage of development, when apposition of the hard tissues of the crown is well advanced, the cervical loop grows to form a double layer of epithelial cells known as 'Hertwig's root sheath'. It is under the influence of this sheath that the roots develop. Frequently one finds in histological sections a few stellate cells sandwiched between the inner and outer epithelia in the root sheath. During development, Hertwig's sheath grows basally between the tooth follicle and the dental papilla and it comes to enclose the papilla except for an opening at its base, known as the 'primary apical foramen' (*Fig. 18.1*). Hence, root morphogenesis is bound up with the dynamic activity of Hertwig's sheath.

At first Hertwig's sheath is angled beneath the dental papilla in which form it has been termed a 'root diaphragm'. It seems likely that the base of the growing dental papilla pushes the root sheath outwards moulding it to the shape of the base of the fibrous follicle. As the major cusps form on the crown of a molariform tooth, the papilla pushes irregularly outwards as a number of lobes. These lobes produce corresponding 'bays' in the outline of the root which surrounds it. The 'bays' correspond in number and location with the definitive roots (*Fig. 18.2*). The tongues of epithelial tissue separating the bays now grow inwards to outline the secondary apical foramina and to fuse near the centre of the crown base: the number of the roots thus corresponds with the number of bays in the root diaphragm. The fact that the outward expansion of the papilla generates bays in the root diaphragm might create the impression that there is no intrinsic growth in the diaphragm. However, although not as abundant as might be expected, mitosis figures are found in the cells of the diaphragm from its inception indicating its growth in area. This growth is masked because the base of the dental papilla is expanding at the same rate as the root diaphragm is growing to surround it. Only in regions where the rate of ectodermal growth is greater than the rate of expansion of the base of the dental papilla can the ectoderm divide the root base into separate root areas.

Each secondary apical foramen will ultimately open at a root apex. Where the tongues of tissue meet, running from near the centre of the crown base to the inner aspect of each root, junction lines form, which may be visible as low dentine ridges on the completed tooth. Local defects may occur along these junction lines to produce pulpo-periodontal canals each containing a blood vessel and a nerve. These are found most

ROOT FORMATION

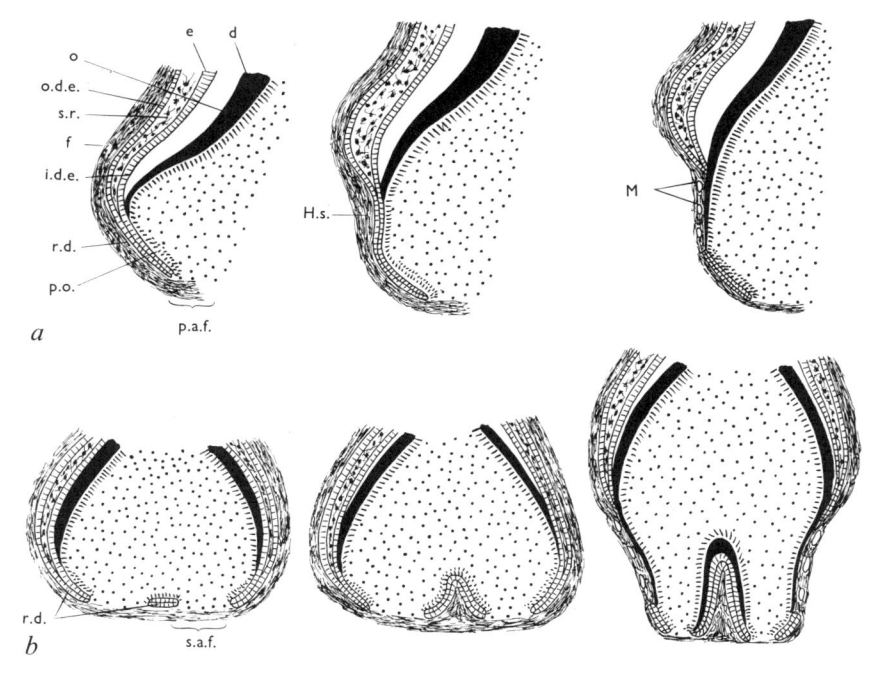

Fig. 18.1. Diagrams of three successive stages in root formation, *a*, in a single-rooted tooth, *b*, in a two-rooted tooth. Not to scale. *d*, dentine; *e*, enamel; *f*, tooth follicle; *H.s.*, Hertwig's root sheath; *i.d.e.*, inner dental epithelium; *M*, Malassez rests; *o*, odontoblasts; *o.d.e.*, outer dental epithelium; *p.a.f.*, primary apical foramen; *p.o.*, differentiating odontoblasts; *r.d.*, epithelial root diaphragm; *s.a.f.*, secondary apical foramen; *s.r.*, stellate reticulum. In *a* there is a single persistent primary apical foramen. In *b* the primary apical foramen is rapidly divided to produce two secondary apical foramina.

commonly in the root bifurcations of deciduous molars. If the adjacent sheaths remain slightly separated in the region of the junction narrow dentine bridges connecting adjacent roots may be formed.

It will be recalled that when discussing the blood supply to the tooth it was shown that vessels entering the dental papilla collect in groups whose number and disposition predict the location of the definitive roots. These groups of vessels lie in the bays in the developing root diaphragm, and the tissue tongues expand inwards between the vessels to unite in the less vascular centre of the crown base.

In single-rooted teeth the procedure is precisely the same but no bays form in the free edge of the root diaphragm, probably due to the absence of developing lobes in the dental papilla. Furthermore, pulpo-periodontal canals are less common in the coronal half of these teeth.

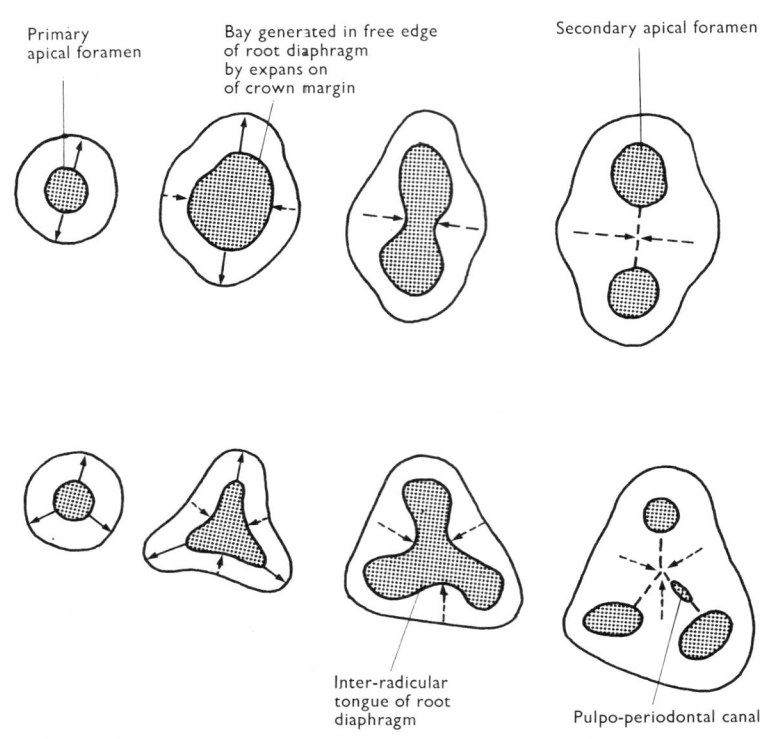

Fig. 18.2. Diagrams showing successive stages in the process of subdivision of the primary apical foramen; as seen from below, producing a two- and a three-rooted tooth. The shaded area represents the papilla seen through the apical foramen. The solid arrows show the direction of expansion of the crown margin. The broken arrows show the direction of growth of the inter-radicular tissue tongues of the root diaphragm. Not to scale.

Once the secondary apical foramina have been delineated in a multi-rooted tooth, a true Hertwig's sheath is present. This continues to grow in a vertical direction. The length of the root is a function of either the degree of intrinsic growth of Hertwig's sheath or of growth of the dental papilla and it is not yet conclusively established which tissue plays the dominant role.

As Hertwig's sheath grows vertically, it induces the differentiation of odontoblasts at the papilla surface. The odontoblasts produce the dentine of the root which lengthens in an apical direction.

After completing its organizing function Hertwig's sheath is involved in the formation of first formed cement (*see* Chapter 17) and then it fragments, with remnants persisting in the adult periodontal ligament as the epithelial cell rests of Malassez. Various functions have been ascribed to these cell rests from time to time, though without any evidence. Histochemical studies reveal the continuing viability of these cells throughout life, albeit in a quiescent state so that the term 'rests' is a reflection of their metabolic state. The following suggestion is offered to explain the fragmentation of Hertwig's root sheath. It was noted that during the formation of the bud, cap and bell stages of tooth development the free margin of the enamel organ (the cervical loop) grows around the expanding dental papilla. It has been demonstrated by serial radiographic examination that the tip of a growing root does not penetrate far into the basally adjacent alveolar bone until the tooth has erupted into the oral cavity and met its opponent (*Fig. 18.3*). Because the tip of the growing root is roughly stationary then so also is the tip of Hertwig's root sheath. In other words Hertwig's root sheath is not growing downwards into the jaw but the root dentine (and enamel) are moving away from it (*Fig. 18.3 a–d*). As the cells of the root sheath proliferate in their continuing attempt to surround the dental papilla they may be pulled towards the oral cavity by the moving root. Because it is being pulled coronally by the lengthening root the proliferating root sheath is prevented from growing round the base of the papilla and sealing the apical foramen. The pull produces tension on the sheet of epithelial cells splitting it into a fenestrated pattern. This may explain why no degeneration of root sheath is seen when it breaks up. When the erupting tooth has met its opponent the lengthening root can no longer slide past the root sheath which will now start to encircle the base of the papilla and complete the formation of the apical foramen of the tooth (*Fig. 18.3e*).

Although in Hertwig's sheath the cell layer nearest the papilla is directly continuous with the inner enamel epithelium over the crown, its cells do not pass through the same cycle of histodifferentiation, nor do they

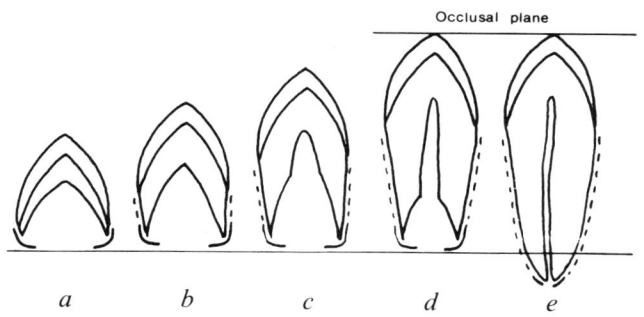

Fig. 18.3. Four stages in the development and eruption of a tooth. During stages *a*, *b*, and *c* the tip of the lengthening root is maintained at the same distance from the lower border of the mandible. Alveolar bone develops around the erupting tooth. While the tooth erupts Hertwig's root sheath is pulled coronally together with the moving root. When the crown meets the opposing tooth the root begins to extend back into the jaw.

normally produce any enamel. The histochemical content of the two cell strata is different. Commonly, however, small enamel pearls are formed on the surface of roots, particularly at the bifurcation of roots. This shows, therefore, that some root-sheath cells are potentially capable of producing enamel. It is well known that coronal odontoblasts differentiate under the influence of the overlying inner dental epithelium. There is no doubt that a similar inductive function is the prime role of Hertwig's sheath.

Unsuccessful attempts have been made to correlate the number and location of the roots with the position of the major cusps on the crown of the molariform tooth. In the late eighteenth century it was suggested that a relationship existed between the pattern of blood vessels supplying the developing tooth and the presence of morphogenetic fields within it. More recently, these fields have been equated with cuspal areas, thought to be controlled by growth centres located within the pulp, under the influence of which specific parts of the crown pattern are generated. Direct evidence of these areas and centres is lacking, but it seems reasonable to expect that each should receive an adequate blood supply via the roots. Hence the number and disposition of the roots would bear a relationship to the number and location of the cuspal areas and growth centres within the papilla, thereby establishing a link between the crown pattern and the root pattern.

REFERENCES AND FURTHER READING

Carlson H. (1944) Studies in the role and amount of eruption in certain human teeth. *Am. J. Orthod.* **30**, 575.

Gaunt W. A. (1960) The vascular supply in relation to the formation of roots on the cheek of the mouse. *Acta Anat.* **43**, 116.

Kenney E. B. and Ramfjord S. P. (1969) Cellular dynamics in root formation of teeth in rhesus monkeys. *J. Dent. Res.* **48**, 114.

Kovacs I. (1971) A systematic description of dental roots. In: Dahlberg A. A. (ed.), *Dental Morphology and Evolution.* Chicago, University of Chicago, p. 211.

Lester K. S. (1969) The incorporation of epithelial cells by cementum. *J. Ultrastruct. Res.* **27**, 63.

Noble H. W., Carmichael A. F. and Rankine D. M. (1962) Electronmicroscopy of human developing dentine. *Arch. Oral Biol.* **7**, 395.

Orban E. and Mueller E. (1929) The development of the bifurcation of multirooted teeth. *J. Am. Dent. Ass.* **16**, 297.

Owens P. D. A. (1972) Light microscope observations on the formation of the layer of Hopewell–Smith in human teeth. *Arch. Oral Biol.* **17**, 1985.

Owens P. D. A. (1974) A light microscopic study of the development of the roots of premolar teeth in dogs. *Arch. Oral Biol.* **20**, 709.

Owens P. D. A. (1976) The root surface in human teeth: a microradiographic study. *J. Anat.* **122**, 389.

Owens, P. D. A. (1980) A light and electron microscopic study of the early stages of root surface formation in molar teeth in the rat. *Arch. Oral Biol.* **24**, 901.

CHAPTER 19

THE PERIODONTIUM

The periodontium is properly described as the supporting apparatus of the tooth consisting of cement, periodontal ligament, alveolar bone, and the dento-gingival junction, the latter consisting of junctional and crevicular epithelia and their supporting connective tissue. Cement, bone and the dento-gingival junction are discussed separately and this chapter deals largely with the periodontal ligament. Even so, the periodontium should always be considered as the functional unit involved in tooth support.

Development

The periodontal ligament is classically described as originating from the dental follicle, that is the mesenchyme between the forming alveolar bone and the developing tooth. However, if the cap and the early bell stages of tooth development are examined carefully it can be seen that the ectomesenchyme of the dental papilla continues around the cervical loop of the dental organ to form an investing layer around the developing tooth (*Fig. 19.1*). As will be described, the tooth's supporting tissues arise from this layer and it is proposed that the term 'follicle' be reserved for it, and it

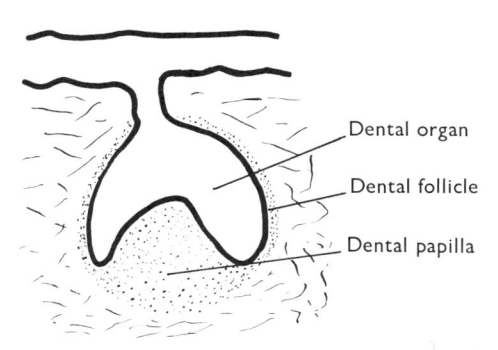

Fig. 19.1. Diagram showing the continuity of the dental papilla with the investing layer around the dental organ.

is so used here. Thus the tooth germ consists of dental organ (the formative organ of enamel), the dental papilla (the formative organ of the dentine-pulp complex) and the dental follicle (the formative organ of tooth support). Over the past few years studies have shown that the cells of the follicle give rise to cementoblasts, fibroblasts and osteoblasts which in turn form cement, periodontal ligament and bone. In fact, apart from the gingival component, cells of the follicle can give rise to the entire periodontium. This was established by dissecting out tooth germs at the bell stage of development from day-old mice, labelling the cells of the investing layer with tritiated thymidine and then implanting these tooth germs subcutaneously in adult mice (*Fig. 19.2*). In this location the tooth germs continue to develop and 3–4 weeks later resemble adequately a tooth. Significantly, cement, periodontal ligament and bone develop in

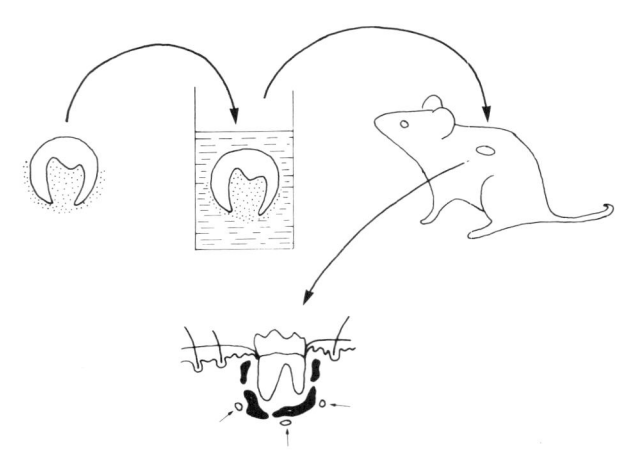

Fig. 19.2. Experimental evidence for the origin of periodontium. A dissected tooth germ is radioactively labelled in a solution of thymidine and implanted beneath the skin of a mouse. The tooth together with periodontal ligament and alveolar bone are all formed. Rejection cells (arrowed) develop on the outer surface of the 'alveolar' bone.

relation to the roots of these subcutaneous teeth. The cementoblasts and ligament fibroblasts are labelled with tritiated thymidine thus establishing their origin from the implanted tooth germ. That the bone cells originated from the same source was established by demonstrating lymphocytes (graft rejection cells) in relation to subcutaneous bone. Interestingly enough in some instances the teeth in this subcutaneous location erupted and established an epithelial attachment. These experiments complement previous *in vitro* studies which showed that when tooth germs are kept in culture for 30 days only a few scattered epithelial and ectomesenchymal cells survive. If these few cells are harvested and transferred to a connective tissue site, such as the base of the mouse tail tendon, they resume their developmental potential and form a tooth with associated cement, periodontal ligament and bone.

More recently some sophisticated experiments have conclusively demonstrated the origin of the tooth's supporting tissues from the dental follicle. Decalcified bone matrix is implanted into muscle or subcutaneous tissue and osteogenic cells differentiate from the local cell population and form bone. When the same material is implanted into the anterior chamber of the eye no bone forms indicating that osteogenic progenitor cells do not exist in this location. However, when a tooth germ is implanted into the anterior chamber of the eye tooth formation continues with the development of its associated supporting tissues, including bone. Significantly in these experiments the dental organ, dental papilla and dental follicle were separated from each other and recombined in various combinations before reimplantation in the eye. Thus, when dental organ and papilla were recombined the tooth and its supporting tissues formed. When dental organ and dental follicle were recombined the results depended upon the age of the implanted tissues. When tissues were obtained from 16-day-old (mouse) embryos, 70 per cent of the implants formed teeth with the full complement of supporting tissues. The same tissues from older embryos resulted in only 15 per cent of the implants forming tooth. From these results it can be concluded that the dental papilla and dental follicle have the same developmental potential early in the ontogeny of the tooth and this is consistent with the assumption that both are derived from the same neural crest line. However, at a specific time during development (after 16 days in the mouse) the follicle becomes determined to form tooth supporting tissue only.

The embryological specificity of the tooth's supporting tissues should dictate thinking about the regeneration and repair of tooth support. For example, it provides a ready explanation why avulsed teeth reimplanted with adherent periodontal ligament more often re-establish an attachment than teeth from which soft tissue has been scraped from the root surface. In the former instance a source of progenitor cells exist, whereas in the latter case ankylosis usually ensues as repair cells come from marrow and deposit bone. In the light of this information one must question the value of osseous grafts around teeth as a clinical procedure to replace attachment lost by periodontal disease. Such grafts may well initiate new bone formation around teeth but there is no evidence that any attachment forms—nor can there be any if no progenitor cells are available.

These types of experiments have been extended a little further. If the supporting tissues of the tooth are formed from the follicle it should be possible to implant tooth germs into bone, rather than into soft connective tissue, and form a true gomphosis if the pre-existing bone fuses with the bone generated by the tooth germ. This has been demonstrated to be the case in the following way. When a hole is drilled in the rodent parietal bone the hole, for some reason, does not fill with bone during repair but instead becomes filled with fibrous tissue. If a tooth germ is placed into a similar hole the tooth continues development and forms its own supporting tissue, including new bone, which fuses with the old parietal bone and a true gomphosis forms. While such accounts may seem to be of no practical importance, and a discussion of the origin of the periodontium academic, information of this nature may well be of future significance in relation to tooth germ transplants.

Structure: Cells

When describing the histology of the periodontal ligament, emphasis is usually placed on the collagen fibre bundles which are so easily distinguished in section. However, it is the cells of the periodontal ligament which make this tissue viable and which are responsible for the architecture of its fibrous component.

The cells of the ligament are preponderantly fibroblasts which are responsible for the formation, maintenance and remodelling of the collagen fibre bundles and their associated ground substance. Also included in the cellular pool of the ligament are the bone-associated cells lining the wall of the alveolus, the cement-associated cells and the epithelial cell rests of Malassez. The latter group of cells are fragmented remains of Hertwig's epithelial root sheath which persist in a form of an epithelial network closer to the root surface than to the bone surface of the alveolus. In man the epithelial cell rests have been shown to be viable in the mature ligament and to have the histochemical and ultrastructural features of resting cells. It has been shown *in vitro* and *in vivo* that they retain their ability to divide and migrate under altered environmental conditions and form the epithelial lining of dental cysts. Other cellular elements in the ligament are associated with the neural and vascular elements.

It is helpful to remember that the tooth in function makes constant demands upon its supporting apparatus which involve the continual adjustment of its structural components. Thus, on the bone surface of the alveolus many states of bone histology occur varying from bone deposition, resorption, to resting bone surface and the histology of the bone-associated cells varies accordingly. It is also now known that the rate of turnover and remodelling of the collagen in the periodontal ligament is exceptionally high, probably higher than anywhere else in the body (for example, in the mouse molar ligament the half-life of the collagen has been demonstrated to be 24 hours!) and this reflects the constant state of flux required by the ligament as it functions. Clearly turnover involves the synthesis and degradation of collagen and the ligament fibroblast is able to synthesize and degrade collagen fibrils simultaneously as described in Chapter 9.

Structure: Fibres

The histology of the main fibre groups of the periodontal ligament is adequately described in the literature and their anatomy is not considered here. Surprisingly, little is known about the development of the principal fibre groups of the periodontal ligament. It has been suggested that the principal oblique fibres are orientated at the time of root development, an arrangement which is initially seen in histological sections as an oblique orientation of fibroblasts and that the fibres they form therefore assume the same orientation. Once formed their orientation is amended by changes in the position of the tooth relative to the alveolar crest as the tooth erupts. Thus, before tooth eruption begins the crest of the alveolar bone is above the cement–enamel junction and all the fibre bundles in the forming ligament are obliquely directed. When the level of the cement–enamel junction coincides with the crest of the alveolus the fibre bundles are aligned horizontally and with further tooth movement become aligned obliquely again, but now in the reverse direction. It seems that only after function do the fibre bundles of the periodontal ligament thicken appreciably.

Supportive Function

The configuration of the oblique fibre bundles suggests that they function as ties uniting the root to the alveolus, and that under load these fibres transmit the force as tension to the alveolar bone. Indeed, the oblique fibres are classically described as having a wavy configuration in the relaxed state but that they straighten out under load. However, there is now a great deal of evidence which shows that this concept is too simplified. For example, if the fibres of the periodontal ligament are cut on the mesial and distal aspects of the tooth, little increase in horizontal mobility occurs, indicating that the fibres are not important in resisting horizontal force. Frequently, when dried skulls are examined, fenestrations in the labial wall of the alveolus not associated with pathological lesions are seen, indicating that a complete bony alveolus is not necessary for tooth support. Under axial load it has been shown that the bony margins of the socket supporting the tooth dilate. If this axial load were converted to tension on the socket wall as suggested by the orientation of the fibres, the reverse would be anticipated.

This finding can be explained if a compressional system, as well as a tensional system, plays a significant part in tooth support. The ligament can be considered as a compressive hydraulic buffer consisting of a vascular component and a tissue fluid component. The suggestion is that under axial compression, the vascular elements are occluded, followed by the displacement of tissue fluid. However, it has been shown that the periodontal vessels of the monkey incisor unexpectedly failed to collapse when measured pressures were applied to the tooth, and it has been suggested that the maintenance of the patency of blood vessels under pressure is a function of the oxytalan fibres found in the periodontal ligament. Oxytalan fibres are considered to be a variant of elastic tissue and have been shown to have distribution within the periodontal ligament closely linked to blood vessels. Thus they are found to run obliquely between vessels and cement, mainly perpendicular to the occlusal plane and at right angles to the direction of the collagen. The insertion of oxytalan fibres into cement implies an anchorage for the vessels which may permit them to accommodate distortion and compression strains. Even though the vessels may remain patent it is still thought the blood is displaced from the system.

The other component of this postulated hydraulic buffer mechanism, the tissue fluid, is considered to be more significant in terms of tooth support. As fluids are incompressible, the cells and extracellular fluid must be displaced if a tooth is pushed into its socket. Where the fluid is displaced is not known; it probably varies with the type of force. If the tooth is subjected to a horizontal force there is some degree of tilt and fluid can be displaced from a region of compression towards a region of tension. Under axial load the fluid can be displaced through the socket wall which is extensively perforated by foramina distributed mainly in the cervical and apical thirds. Also the outward displacement of the socket margin under axial compression suggests tissue fluid displacement towards the rim of the socket. In this case the collagen fibres might act as ties preventing overdilatation of the socket.

Recently the results of some experiments of measuring axial displacement have expanded and unified the concept of ligament function. The suggestion is that there is a sequence of three basic positioning mechanisms within the periodontium. First, there is a simple short-term recoil of tissues and a return of blood to the system following normal chewing. Second, if a chewing sequence involves a longer succession of chewing thrusts it is suggested that the water bound to the ground substance is released and transported away. Recovery would be medium term involving repolymerization of the ground substance and rebinding of the intercellular fluid.

The third positioning mechanism is achieved by turnover of the collagen fibre bundles which controls the position of the tooth within its socket and occurs in response to long-term forces, such as a persistent force provided by orthodontic therapy.

When the periodontium is considered it is usually thought of in relation to a single tooth. However, recent studies have indicated further connections between the periodontium of adjacent teeth in addition to the long-established trans-septal fibre system. Thus gingival fibres have been described running from one tooth to the adjacent tooth, as have ligament fibres passing through septal bone. It is most likely that some of these fibres are responsible for approximal (mesial or distal) drift, that is movement of the teeth to maintain approximal contact. Thus it has been shown that teeth, isolated from masticatory forces and from the cheeks, tongue and lips, drift continuously and that, if the trans-septal group of fibres is severed, a reduction in drift occurs.

Another controversial feature of the anatomy of the periodontium is the so-called intermediate plexus. The concept here is that in the middle region of the ligament the collagen of the principal fibre bundles is constantly being broken and reformed to permit tooth movement in an occlusal direction. It has been argued that the histological demonstration of an intermediate plexus in longitudinal sections of teeth in situ may be due to the fact that fibres are cut obliquely in the middle of the ligament and radially towards its periphery. No intermediate plexus can be demonstrated in transverse sections through the ligament. However, although the bright field light microscopic appearance of an intermediate plexus may be artefactual, polarized light microscopy indicates that the collagen fibres in the central zone of the ligament are less mature. Also, in experimental avitaminosis C, which interferes with collagen production, the intermediate zone of the ligament shows the greatest degree of disruption which suggests that this is the most active site of collagen synthesis. Radiobiological studies have not helped as much as might have been anticipated. Studies using radioactive proline have not demonstrated remodelling in a clearcut intermediate zone. Instead a fairly even pattern of remodelling occurs with the lowest activity towards the cement surface of the tooth.

However, the above studies indicate that the periodontium has an exceptionally high rate of remodelling and turnover, probably the highest of any connective tissue, and that this involves the degradation and synthesis of collagen. Electron microscopic and histochemical examination of the periodontal ligament has shown that its fibroblasts are capable of phagocytosing and degrading collagen as well as synthesizing this material. Furthermore, these ultrastructural studies provide no evidence for an intermediate plexus. The fact that ligament fibroblasts are able to synthesize and degrade collagen explains how adaptation of ligament might take place during eruption, function and tooth movement.

Sensory Function

The periodontal ligament, in addition to its supportive role, also has an important role as a sensory receptor; a grain of sand in a sandwich is readily detected by receptors in the periodontal ligament. The periodontal ligament contains nerve fibres running from the apical region towards the gingival margin which are joined by fibres entering the ligament laterally through the foramina of the socket wall. The latter divide into two, with one branch running apically and the other gingivally. The manner in which these nerve fibres terminate has been clarified recently. Some fibres are thought to terminate as free unmyelinated nerve endings and to be associated with pain. Others terminate in specific mechano-receptors and two types have been described possibly associated with the recognition of elastic deformation and with the recognition of viscous transmission of pressure. It has also been suggested that these structural variations of mechano-receptors are not really important and that it is their spatial arrangement within the ligament that is the determining factor in their response characteristics. The blood supply of the ligament is dealt with in Chapter 8.

REFERENCES AND FURTHER READING

Anderson D. J., Hannam A. G. and Mathews B. (1970) Sensory mechanisms in mammalian teeth and their supporting structures. *Physiol. Rev.* **50**, 171.

Atkinson M. E. (1972) The development of the mouse molar periodontium. *J. Periodont. Res.* **7**, 255.

Beertsen W. and Snijder J. (1970) A comparative study on the histological structure of the periodontal membranes of teeth with a continuous and with a non-continuous eruption. *Neth. Dent. J.* **77**, 24.

Bernick S. (1960) The organization of the periodontal membrane fibres of the developing molars of rats. *Neth. Dent. J.* **2**, 57.

Bevelander G. and Nakahara H. (1968) The fine structure of the human periodontal ligament. *Anat. Rec.* **162**, 313.

Carmichael G. G. (1968) Observations with the light microscope on the distribution and connections of the oxytalan fibre of the lower jaw of the mouse. *Arch. Oral Biol.* **13**, 765.

Carmichael G. G. and Fullmer H. M. (1966) The fine structure of the oxytalan fibre. *J. Cell Biol.* **28**, 33.

Cohn S. A. (1972a) A re-examination of Sharpey's fibres in alveolar bone of the mouse. *Arch. Oral Biol.* **17**, 255.

Cohn S. A. (1972b) A re-examination of Sharpey's fibres in alveolar bone of the marmoset (*Saguinus fuscicollis*). *Arch. Oral Biol.* **17**, 261.

Coolidge E. D. (1937) The thickness of the human periodontal membrane. *J. Am. Dent. Assoc.* **24**, 1260.

Eccles J. D. (1959) Studies on the development of the periodontal membrane: the principal fibres of the molar teeth. *Dent. Practnr Dent. Rec.* **10**, 31.

Eley B. M. and Harrison J. D. (1975) Intracellular collagen fibrils in the periodontal ligament of man. *J. Periodont. Res.* **10**, 168.

Freeman E. and Ten Cate A. R. (1971) Development of the periodontium: an electron microscope study. *J. Periodont.* **42**, 387.

Freeman E., Ten Cate A. R. and Dickinson J. (1975) Development of a gomphosis by tooth germ implants in the parietal bone of the mouse. *Arch. Oral Biol.*, **20**, 139.

Fullman H. M., Sheetz J. H. and Narkates A. J. (1974) Oxytalan connective tissue fibres: a review. *J. Oral Pathol.* **3**, 291.

Furstman L. and Bernick S. (1965) Early development of the periodontal membrane. *Am. J. Orthod.* **51**, 482.

Garant P. R. (1976) Collagen resorption by fibroblasts. A theory of fibroblastic maintenance of periodontal ligament. *J. Periodont.* **47**, 380.

Grant D. A. and Bernick S. (1972) Formation of the periodontal ligament. *J. Periodont.* **43**, 17.

Grant D. A., Bernick S., Levy B. M. et al. (1972) A comparative study of periodontal ligament development in teeth with and without predecessors in marmosets. *J. Periodont.* **43**, 162.

Griffin C. J. and Harris R. (1967) The fine structure of the developing human periodontium. *Arch. Oral Biol.* **12**, 971.

Griffin C. J. and Harris R. (1968) Unmyelinated nerve endings in the periodontal membrane of human teeth. *Arch. Oral Biol.* **13**, 1207.

Hannam A. G. (1976) Periodontal mechanoreceptors. In: Anderson D. J. and Matthews B. (ed.), *Mastication*. Wright, Bristol, p. 43.

Harris, R. (1975) Innervation of the human periodontium. *Monogr. Oral Sci.* **41**, 27. Basel, Karger.

Hoffman R. L. (1960) Formation of periodontal tissues around subcutaneously transplanted hamster molars. *J. Dent. Res.* **39**, 781.

Melcher A. H. and Bowen W. H. (1969) *The Biology of the Periodontium*. New York, Academic.

Parfitt G. J. (1960) Measurement of the physiological mobility of individual teeth in an axial direction. *J. Dent. Res.* **39**, 608.

Picton D. C. A. (1965) On the part played by the socket in tooth support. *Arch. Oral Biol.* **10**, 945.

Picton D. C. A. (1967) Dimensional changes in the periodontal membrane of monkeys. *Arch. Oral Biol.* **12**, 1635.

Simpson H. E. (1966) The innervation of the periodontal membrane as observed by the apoxestic technique. *J. Periodont.* **37**, 374.

Sims M. R. (1973) Oxytalan fiber system of molars in the mouse mandible. *J. Dent. Res.* **52**, 797.

Sodek J. (1977) A comparison of the rates of synthesis and turnover of collagen and non-collagen proteins in adult rat periodontal tissues and skin using a microassay. *Arch. Oral Biol.* **22**, 655.

Sodek J., Brunette D. M., Feng I. et al. (1977) Collagen synthesis is a major component of protein synthesis in the periodontal ligament in various species. *Arch. Oral Biol.* **22**, 647.

Ten Cate A. R. (1966) The development of the periodontium. In: Melcher A. H. and Bowen W. H. (ed.), *Biology of the Periodontium*. London, Academic p. 53.

Ten Cate A. R. (1972a) Cell division and periodontal ligament formation in the mouse. *Arch. Oral Biol.* **17**, 1781.

Ten Cate A. R. (1972b) Developmental aspects of the periodontium. In: Slavkin H. C. and Bavetta L. A. (ed.), *Developmental Aspects of Oral Biology*. London, Academic, p. 309.

Ten Cate A. R. and Mills C. (1972) The development of the periodontium: the origin of alveolar bone. *Anat. Rec.* **173**, 69.

Ten Cate A. R., Mills. C. and Solomon G. (1971) The development of the periodontium: a transplantation and autoradiographic study. *Anat. Rec.* **170**, 365.

Tonge C. H. (1963) The development and arrangement of the dental follicle. *Trans. Eur. Orth. Soc.* p. 118.

Wills D. J. and Picton D. C. A (1978) Changes in the mobility and resting position of incisor teeth in macaque monkeys. *Arch. Oral Biol* **23**, 225.

Wills D. J. and Picton D. C. A. (1981) Changes in the force–intrusion relationship of the tooth with its resting position in macaque monkeys. *Arch. Oral Biol.* **26**, 827–829.

Wills D. J., Picton D. C. A. and Davies W. I. R. (1976) A study of the fluid systems of the periodontium in macaque monkeys. *Arch. Oral Biol.* **21**, 175.

Wills D. J., Picton D. C. A. and Davies W. I. R. (1978) The intrusion of the tooth for different loading rates. *J. Biomechanics* **11**, 429.

Yoshikawa D. K. and Kollar E. J. (1981) Recombination experiments on the odontogenic roles of mouse dental papilla and dental sac tissues in ocular grafts. *Arch. Oral Biol.* **26**, 303.

CHAPTER 20

PHYSIOLOGICAL TOOTH MOVEMENT

Teeth can, and do, move in the bony jaws—but how they move is an intriguing biological problem.

When tooth movement in non-mammalian vertebrates is studied where tooth succession, and therefore tooth movement, is often a continuous process, it is clear that the operation of a couple of factors—displacement of the entire tooth and growth of the tooth—results in the movement of teeth. The relative contribution of each factor seems to vary in the vertebrate classes. For example, in elasmobranchs tooth displacement is the significant component achieving the final functional position of the tooth, whereas in reptiles axial growth of the tooth predominates.

Interestingly, in the light of what follows when mammalian tooth movement is discussed, it has been observed that in many instances in non-mammalian vertebrates a system of fibres exist which link the erupting tooth to surrounding hard tissue. Thus, in elasmobranchs and crocodilians, such fibres come to form the attachment apparatus of the tooth. In teleosts these fibres form a follicle which is lost when the teeth come into function and in lizards an ill-defined band of connective tissue can be recognized at the time the tooth movement is taking place, and the tentative suggestion has been made that these fibre systems exert some form of traction on the tooth.

In mammals teeth are socketed and attached to the bone of the jaw by a periodontal ligament but tooth movement is also brought about by a combination of tooth displacement and tooth growth.

In man tooth movement is, for descriptive purposes, divided into pre-eruptive, eruptive and post-eruptive stages, with eruptive tooth movement defined as the axial movement of the tooth which brings the crown of the tooth from its developmental position within the bone of the jaw to its functional position in the occlusal plane. Its commencement can be roughly equated with the onset of root formation.

PRE-ERUPTIVE TOOTH MOVEMENT

The movements a tooth germ makes within the developing and growing jaws before it begins its eruptive movement seem to be extensive as, for example, the migration of the permanent first pre-molar tooth germ from the lingual aspect of the crown of the deciduous molar tooth germ to a position between its roots. But it must be remembered that these movements may be exaggerated because of the shift of landmarks in a rapidly expanding situation so that, in the example cited above, not only is the jaw increasing in height and in length but the deciduous tooth is moving significantly in its eruptive phase. The associated permanent successional tooth germ is of course in its pre-eruptive phase.

Histologically pre-eruptive tooth movement has been described in terms of bony remodelling, and of recording areas of bone deposition and resorption on the crypt walls. But this exercise only gives information about directions of tooth movement. It does not explain how such movement is achieved as it is not known whether the demonstrated bony remodelling is the cause of, or is a response to, tooth movement.

ERUPTIVE TOOTH MOVEMENT

While eruptive tooth movement has been defined as movement in an axial plane, it must be understood that as the tooth is erupting it may also be moving in planes other than axial associated with growth of the jaws. Eruptive movements have attracted much attention but, as yet, no definitive explanation of the forces that bring them about has been provided. Detailed descriptions exist of the histological changes which occur at the time of tooth eruption in the tissues of the tooth (root formation: Chapter 18), its follicle (formation of the periodontal ligament: Chapter 19) and the overlying connective tissue and epithelium (development of the dento-gingival junction: Chapter 21) and these chapters should be referred to as the theories of tooth eruption are discussed.

Several theories of tooth eruption exist involving the separate tissues of the dento-alveolar complex. Evidence to support four theories consistently appears and it is most likely that the mechanism for eruption can be explained by one or a combination of these theories. The theories implicate proliferation of the cells involved in tooth growth; pressure generated by vascular tissues; a contractile element within the periodontal ligament and bony remodelling.

Bony Remodelling

Bony remodelling of the jaws has been linked with tooth eruption. It has been suggested that the inherent growth pattern of the mandible and maxilla moves teeth by selective deposition and resorption of bone in the immediate neighbourhood of the tooth. Elegant and careful studies with tetracyclines as bone markers disprove this suggestion. Tetracyclines become incorporated in newly formed bone and can be identified in sections due to their fluorescent properties. With the onset of tooth eruption bone is resorbed at the base of the socket. However, this is followed by deposition of the bone on the socket floor. Measurements show that the amount of bone deposited, plus the amount of root growth, together equal the distance that the tooth moves, which is scarcely surprising. However, some workers seem to consider that this implicates bone growth with tooth eruption, despite the initial resorption of bone as the tooth begins to move in an occlusal direction. It is more likely that the later deposition of bone is an infilling after the tooth has moved; it is an effect, not a cause, of eruption.

In spite of persistent evidence that bony remodelling is a response to tooth movement and therefore cannot be used as evidence to support an inherent growth pattern within the jaws, there is some experimental evidence which cannot be ignored and suggests some predetermination for tooth movement. If successional tooth germs are either 'wired down' or enucleated surgically, an eruptive pathway still forms through the bone with osteoclasts widening the gubernacular canal in the absence of an erupting tooth. These observations have been generally ignored in discussions on tooth eruption.

Cell Proliferation and Root Foundation

Cell proliferation brings about root formation. Although attempts have been made to interfere with cellular proliferation no single cell population (for example, pulp fibroblasts, root sheath cells or periodontal fibroblasts) can be destroyed without interfering with other cells. Therefore although cell proliferation appears to be necessary to maintain normal tooth eruption, the force which this activity generates, either directly or indirectly, is not known.

When root formation *in toto* is considered, including epithelial proliferation, dentine deposition and pulpal proliferation, it has been suggested that increase in the length of the forming root provides the eruptive force by pushing against a structure termed the 'cushion hammock ligament'. This structure was described as passing from one side of the socket, under the root apex, to the opposite wall of the socket and its function was thought to be to convert the downward thrust exerted by the growing root into a pull on the socket wall. It has now been clearly demonstrated that this structure is an artefact and is really a pulp-delineating membrane with no connection to the bone of the socket wall. Furthermore, it is known that eruptive tooth movement occurs in teeth whose apices have closed and where presumably cell proliferation has ceased.

Fluid Pressure

Some elegant measurements have been made of tissue fluid pressures below and above erupting, but as yet unerupted, teeth in the dog. These have demonstrated that there is a pressure differential of about 15 mmHg, which is more than sufficient to account for eruption. Theoretically it seems possible that by opening precapillary sphincters at the base of an erupting tooth the tissue fluid pressure in this region could be increased to the extent that sufficient pressure would be generated to push the tooth out of the socket. In a very different situation, everyone is aware of the pressure which can be generated within a boil in the skin before it 'bursts'.

Experimental interference with mechanisms controlling the calibre of blood vessels affects eruption. Thus, vaso-active drugs significantly increase the rate of tooth eruption. Cervical sympathectomy and stimulation of the cervical sympathetic trunk also affect the eruption rate consistent with a haemodynamic hypothesis for tooth eruption. However, the possibility always remains that metabolic changes resulting from experimentally induced changes in local vascularity affect other systems involved in tooth eruption.

Mitigating against the theory of vascular pressure and cell proliferation/root growth are experiments undertaken with the continuously erupting rodent incisor. Many investigations into tooth eruption have made use of this tooth which is permitted to erupt unimpeded by constantly removing the erupted tip of the tooth. While it could be argued that the mechanism for eruption of the very specialized rodent incisor may be unlike that of other teeth there are sufficient parallels, not discussed here, to validate the use of this tooth for inquiry into tooth eruption in general.

Periodontal Ligament

The experiments referred to involve surgical interference with the growing root of the tooth. In one set of experiments (*Fig. 20.1*) the proliferating dental organ and dental papilla of the continuously growing lower incisor of the rat were removed. This eliminated any eruptive force which might have been contributed by cellular proliferation in the forming root. After this procedure the tooth continued to erupt at its normal rate until, because there was no formation of new tissues, the tooth was exfoliated. The fact that the only unoperated dental tissue remaining in this experiment was the periodontal ligament suggests that it provided the force for eruption, perhaps by 'pulling' the tooth out of the socket. However, it could be argued that the inflammatory response to surgical interference led to an accumulation of tissue fluid behind the erupting tooth, and that this fluid, under pressure, was responsible for pushing the tooth out of its socket. Against this interpretation it was argued that if tissue fluid pressure had built up behind the erupting tooth it would have pushed fluid out of the exposed pulp canal (the incisal edge of the tooth was continually cut away to allow unimpeded eruption) (*Fig. 20.1c*). But it

PHYSIOLOGICAL TOOTH MOVEMENT

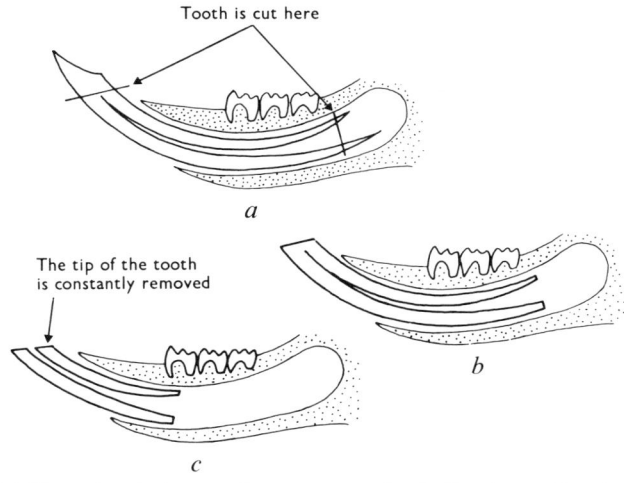

Fig. 20.1. The rodent incisor continues to erupt after its forming end has been surgically removed. The incisal edge of the tooth is constantly removed in order to allow it to erupt more rapidly.

is possible that the exposed, empty, pulp chamber was blocked by clotted inflammatory exudate.

To investigate the above problem further, the dental organ from the labial side of a rodent incisor was removed, thereby preventing any further development of the labial side of the tooth (*Fig. 20.2*). Ultimately, only the newly developed lingual side of the tooth, consisting of dentine and

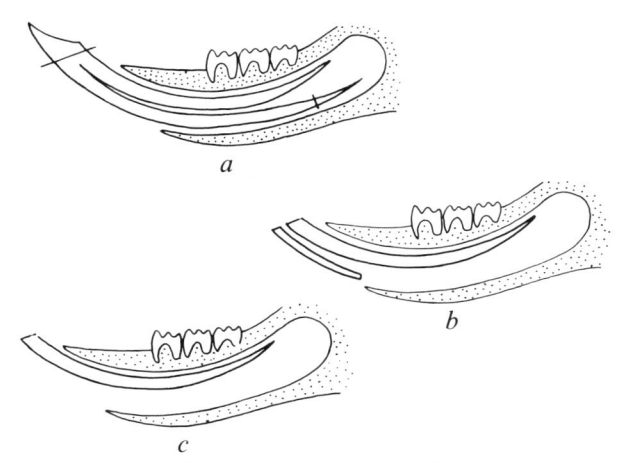

Fig. 20.2. The buccal side of the developing end of a rodent incisor is removed. The isolated lingual side continues to develop and erupt.

cement, remained (*Fig. 20.2c*); and this continued to erupt. It is argued that this fragment is pulled out by some force in the periodontal ligament.

Thus, over the past decade most investigative studies have focused attention on the periodontal ligament as the tissue in which the force moving teeth resides and either the cells of the ligament or the extracellular collagen are thought to provide the force for tooth movement. Collagen is formed and destroyed continuously in the ligament. The collagen macromolecules secreted by the fibroblasts are initially arranged in a random fashion in the extracellular compartment. When these macromolecules become ordered to form collagen fibres, there is a decrease in entropy and this decrease in disorder must provide a force along the axis of the orientating fibres to prevent the macromolecules from returning to their disordered state and this force might move teeth. A reasonable analogy here is a stretched elastic band. When stretched the molecules are in an orderly state (decreased entropy) and there is a contractile force as the molecules try to assume a more disordered state.

Experiments where collagen formation in the ligament is interrupted, for example by denying vitamin C essential for collagen synthesis to the ligament fibroblasts, or administering lathyrogens which prevent the formation of cross-linkages between the collagen molecules, result in disturbance of the normal architecture of the ligament and a retardation of the eruption rate. Significantly in such experiments root formation is not affected and the growing root impinges on the floor of the socket with resorption of the bone and buckling of the root. Also growth of Hertwig's root sheath is undisturbed and the predentine of the root, the pulpal tissue, and the vascular elements appear normal. Thus experimental prevention of normal collagen formation in the ligament apparently prevents tooth eruption and would seem to implicate collagen synthesis as a prime mover of the tooth. In spite of these experiments, much resistance has occurrred to the notion that collagen synthesis *per se* is the cause of tooth eruption. This is because there was some confusing evidence concerning (1) the lathyrogenic effect related to dose response and (2) a false suggestion that collagen synthesis involved dehydration and a 10 per cent reduction in the length of the collagen fibril. In summary, there is no doubt that when collagen synthesis is interfered with in the periodontal ligament a consequence is a change in the rate of tooth eruption. But this does not mean that synthesis of collagen generates a force. For example, it can be argued that the cells of the ligament provide the contractile force and exert this force by pulling on collagen fibre bundles. Clearly if the bundles were disorganized, any eruptive force residing in cells could not take effect. Although there is no evidence that a contractile force existing in fibroblasts is expressed in this way the example is given to illustrate the difficulty of pinpointing the force which moves teeth.

Because there is a contractile mechanism associated with scar tissue formation, and because it is known that the contraction is brought about by modulated fibroblasts which have some structural features and similar pharmacological responses to smooth muscle cells, a search for similar modulated fibroblasts (called myofibroblasts) in the periodontal ligament has been undertaken. To date, no convincing evidence has been presented to confirm or deny the existence of myofibroblasts in this location. While reports of some of the histological features associated with myofibroblasts have occurred, such as the presence of microtubules, microfilaments and cell-to-cell contacts, it has been pointed out that such features may well be associated with other cellular function such as, in the case of microtubules, pinocytosis or exocytosis. The demonstration of contractile proteins such as actin or myosin in ligament fibroblasts is essential if any credence is to be given to the idea that fibroblast contraction moves teeth.

In summary then there is, as yet, no proof that the fibroblast provides the force for tooth eruption. Yet this cell is important for the process of tooth eruption for it has the ability to remodel ligament collagen rapidly and this explains how the ligament can support the tooth in the jaw and at the same time permit eruptive movements.

POST-ERUPTIVE TOOTH MOVEMENTS

Such movements fall into three groupings associated with (1) maintaining the position of the tooth as the jaw grows, especially in height (2) compensating for occlusal wear and, finally, (3) compensating for interproximal wear.

Although at about the age of 12–13 the final arch width in the canine, premolar and molar regions is fixed there is a continued increase in height of the jaws until the end of the second decade. As the jaws increase in height there is a corresponding repositioning of the tooth socket achieved by bony deposition at the alveolar crest and on the floor of the socket. This bony remodelling probably reflects an 'infilling effect' after normal eruptive movement has kept the tooth in position as the height of the jaw changes. Interestingly, this axial movement takes place after the apices of the roots of the erupting teeth have closed and is evidence to discount root growth and cell proliferation as providing the force for axial tooth movement.

Similarly, it is more likely that the same axial movement compensates for occlusal wear rather than, as has been claimed by some, by the continuous deposition of cement around the apices of the roots.

Mesial Drift

Mesial, or approximal, drift is important in the maintenance of normal arch contour and relationships and, when disturbed, results in the crowding of teeth, an increased rate of bone loss in periodontal disease and in the development of the myo-fascial pain dysfunction syndrome. No dispute exists that movement in this plane occurs and indeed such movement was commented upon by John Hunter in the eighteenth century. How this drift is achieved has, however, been extensively debated with participants assuming one position or another. As so often is the case, it is now being appreciated that the cause of mesial drift may well be multifactorial. Some theories advanced to explain mesial drift include (1) an anterior component of occlusal force, (2) soft tissue pressures and (3) contraction of the trans-septal ligament between teeth.

The anterior component of force originates when teeth come into occlusion with the summation of cuspal planes and the mesial inclination of the teeth resulting in the resolution of the biting force into an anterior component. There is no doubt that such a force exists and a simple experiment such as showing that it takes more force to remove a steel strip between clenched teeth than from unclenched jaws demonstrates this. Arguments against this force being the cause of mesial drift include the fact that teeth are only infrequently clenched together and that the incisor teeth are inclined labially—not mesially—and therefore would move in a different plane. In fact, imbrication of the incisors is not an uncommon clinical condition and it has been argued that a force emanating distally would indeed move incisors mesially because of the billiard ball effect (*see Fig. 20.3*). More persuasive arguments against an anterior component of

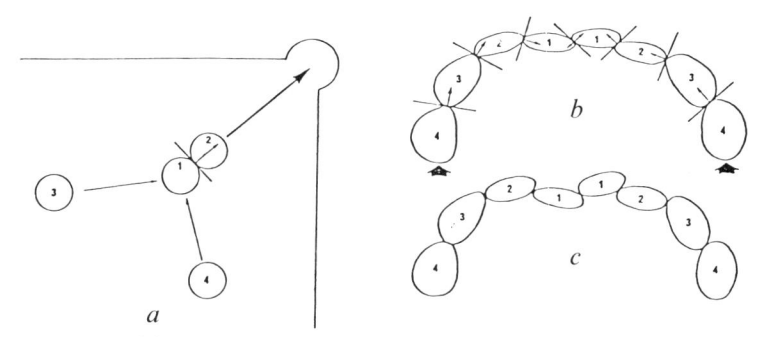

Fig. 20.3. Billiard ball analogy. *a,* If the centres of two touching balls (1 and 2) are in line with a pocket, no matter in what direction (e.g. from 3 or 4) ball 1 is struck, ball 2 enters the pocket. It travels in a direction at right angles to the common tangent between balls 1 and 2. *b.* There is slight imbrication of the central and lateral incisors (1 and 2) in a young dentition. The anterior component of force (large arrows) drives the first premolars (4) forward against the canines (3). From the billiard ball analogy the canines and incisors all move in directions at right angles to common tangents drawn through their contact points (small arrows). This leads to the marked imbrication shown in an older dentition (*c*). From a discussion by Osborn J. (1976). In: Poole D. F. G. and Stack M. V. (ed.), *The Eruption and Occlusion of Teeth.* Colston Papers, No. 27. London Butterworths.

force causing mesial drift come from the results of experiments where this force is eliminated by removing teeth from the opposing arch. Such a procedure does not prevent migration of teeth.

Soft tissue pressure, that is from the cheeks and tongue, has also been suggested as a factor capable of causing mesial drift. Experiments where an acrylic dome was constructed over teeth thereby eliminating soft tissue pressures show that mesial drift still occurs, suggesting that soft tissue pressure does not have a major role, if any, in creating mesial drift. Soft tissue pressure though does influence tooth position even if it is not the cause of mesial drift.

A series of experiments designed to test the hypothesis that contraction of the trans-septal ligament between teeth not only maintains teeth in position but accounts for mesial drift give results apparently confirming the hypothesis. Thus, cutting or scraping the trans-septal fibres at frequent intervals drastically reduces or prevents the drift of teeth. When molar teeth are divided through the bifurcation the two halves separate rapidly if the trans-septal fibres are not cut or removed. These experiments apparently demonstrate that teeth are joined together by a trans-septal fibre system which is under tension, and a final experiment in this series showed that when a break occurs in the system, the teeth posterior to the break do not migrate mesially until repair has taken place. Further evidence that the trans-septal system is an active system comes from radiobiological studies where it has been shown that the ligament, which in histological section seems static, turns over and, furthermore, this rate of turnover increases during orthodontic tooth movement.

Recently a simple, but elegant, experiment has been performed which indicated that the cause of mesial drift is multifactorial. Using monkeys as the experimental animal, the first molars on both sides of the arch were allowed to migrate by removing the approximal contacts, and also by grinding the disto-occlusal surfaces of the second premolars in the upper jaw and the mesio-occlusal surfaces of the second molars in the lower jaw. The first molars on one side were ground out of occlusal contact, while the molars of the contralateral side were untouched. This experimental design is illustrated in *Fig. 20.4*. As a result of these procedures, teeth drifted both in and out of occlusion but the rate of drift was markedly faster on the side where the teeth were in occlusion. The conclusion drawn was that functional occlusion does play an important role in mesial drift but that drift is in response to multiple factors. This was confirmed in another series of experiments which showed that experimental occlusal angulation of teeth in favour of mesial drift caused an increase in the rate of mesial drift, while occlusal modification designed to decrease drift did so. Even so it still seems that traction has a greater influence on tooth position than biting force.

Another way to attempt an analysis of mesial drift is to examine dentitions with ankylosed teeth and use these as fixed reference points.

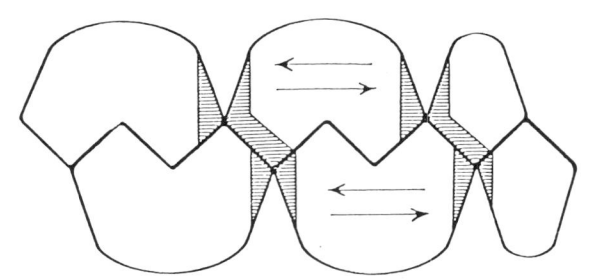

Fig. 20.4. The shaded areas indicate where tissue was removed to facilitate drift. On the other side the molars were ground out of occlusion. From the work of van Beek H. (1976), quoted in a discussion on tooth migration. In: Poole D. F. G. and Stack M. V. (ed.), *The Eruption and Occlusion of Teeth.* Colston Papers, No. 27. London, Butterworths, p. 221.

When this is done, it can be demonstrated that mesial drift can be broken down into two components—there is forward movement of the posterior teeth to close up spacing brought about by interdental attrition, and there is forward movement of the whole arch which can occur without a drive from the back of the arch, although such a force may normally contribute. Clearly the explanation of mesial drift is not yet fully elucidated but, whatever the forces may be, the important factor permitting the expression of these forces applied to teeth is the amazing plasticity of the tissues of the dento-alveolar complex.

REFERENCES AND FURTHER READING

Beertsen W., Everts V. and van der Hoff A. (1974) Fine structure of fibroblasts in the periodontal ligament of the rat incisor and their possible role in tooth eruption. *Arch Oral Biol.* **19**, 1087.

Berkovitz B. K. B. (1971) The effect of root transection and partial root resection on the unimpeded eruption rate of the rat incisor. *Arch. Oral Biol.* **16**, 1033.

Berkovitz B. K. B. (1971) The healing process in the incisor tooth socket of the rat following root resection and exfoliation. *Arch. Oral Biol.* **16**, 1045.

Berkovitz B. K. B. (1972) The effect of preventing eruption on the proliferative basal tissues of the rat lower incisor. *Arch. Oral Biol.* **17**, 1279.

Berkovitz B. K. B. (1975) Mechanisms of tooth eruption. In: Lavelle C. L. B. (ed.), *Applied Physiology of the Mouth.* Bristol, Wright, p. 99.

Berkovitz B. K. B. and Thomas N. R. (1969) Unimpeded eruption in the root resected lower incisor of the rat with a preliminary note on root transection. *Arch. Oral Biol.* **14**, 771.

Bien S. M. (1966) Fluid dynamic mechanisms which regulate tooth movement. In: Staple P. H. (ed.), *Advances in Oral Biology*, Vol. 2. London, Academic, p.173.

Bjork A. E. and Skieller V. (1972) Facial development and tooth eruption. An implant study at the age of puberty. *Am. J. Orthodont.* **62**, 339.

Brash J. C. (1926) The growth of the alveolar bone and its relation to the movements of the teeth, including eruption. *Dent. Rec.* **46**, 641; **47**, 1, 175.

Brash J. C. (1928) The growth of the alveolar bone and its relation to the movements of the teeth, including eruption. *Int. J. Orthodont. Oral Surg. Radiogr.* **14**, 196, 283, 398, 487, 494.

Bryer L. W. (1957) An experimental evaluation of physiology of tooth eruption. *Int. Dent. J.* **7**, 432.

Cahill D. R. (1970) The histology and rate of tooth eruption with and without temporary impaction in the dog. *Anat. Rec.* **166**, 225.

Cahill D. R. (1974) Histological changes in the bony crypt and gubernacular canal of erupting permanent premolars during deciduous premolar exfoliation in beagles. *J. Dent. Res.* **53**, 786.

Carlson H. (1944) Studies in the role and amount of eruption in certain human teeth. *Am. J. Orthod.* **30**, 575.

Carollo D. A., Hoffman R. L. and Brodie A. G. (1971) Histology and function of the dental gubernacular cord. *Angle Orthodont.* **41**, 300.

Constant T. E. (1900) The eruption of the teeth. *Int. Dent. Congr.* **2**, 180.

Enlow D. H. and McNamara J. A., Jr (1973) Varieties of *in vivo* tooth movements. *Angle Orthodont.* **43**, 216.

Jenkins G. N. (1978) *The Physiology of the Mouth*, 4th ed. Oxford, Blackwell Scientific Publications.

Magnusson B. (1968) Tissue changes during molar tooth eruption. *Trans. R. Sch. Dent. Stockholm*, **13**, 1.

Main J. H. P. (1965) A histological survey of the hammock ligament. *Arch. Oral Biol.* **10**, 343.

Main J. H. P. and Adams D. (1966) Experiments on the rat incisor into the cellular proliferation and blood pressure theories of tooth eruption. *Arch. Oral Biol.* **11**, 163.

Manson J. D. (1963a) A study of bone changes associated with tooth eruption. *Proc. R. Soc. Med.* **56**, 515.

Manson J. D. (1963b) Passive eruption. *Dent. Practnr Dent. Rec.* **14**, 2.

Manson J. D. (1967) Bone changes associated with tooth eruption. In: *The Mechanisms of Tooth Support*. A symposium, Oxford, 6–8 July 1965. Bristol, Wright.

Moss J. P. (1976) A review of the theories of approximal migration of teeth. In: Poole D. F. G. and Stack M. V. *The Eruption and Occlusion of Teeth*. Colston Papers, No. 27. London, Butterworths, p. 205.

Moss J. P. and Picton D. C. A. (1967) Experimental mesial drift in adult monkeys (*Macaca irus*). *Arch. Oral Biol.* **12**, 1313.

Moss J. P. and Picton D. C. A. (1970) Mesial drift of teeth in adult monkeys (*Macaca irus*) when forces from the cheeks and tongue had been eliminated. *Arch. Oral Biol.* **15**, 979.

Moss J. P. and Picton D. C. A. (1974) The effect on approximal drift of cheek teeth of dividing mandibular molars of adult monkeys (*Macaca irus*). *Arch. Oral Biol.* **19**, 1211.

Ness A. R. (1964) Movement and forces in tooth eruption. In: Staple P. H. (ed.), *Advances in Oral Biology*, Vol. 1. London, Academic, p. 33.

Ness A. R. (1967) Eruption—a review. In: *The Mechanisms of Tooth Support*, A symposium, Oxford, 6–8 July 1965. Bristol, Wright, p. 84.

Osborn J. W. (1961) An investigation into the interdental forces occuring between the teeth of the same arch during clenching the jaws. *Arch. Oral Biol.* **5**, 202.

Picton D. C. A. (1969) The effect of external forces in the periodontium. In: Melcher A. H. and Bowen W. H. (ed.), *Biology of the Periodontium*. New York, Academic, p. 363.

Picton D. C. A. and Moss J. P. (1973) The part played by the transseptal fibre system in experimental approximal drift of the cheek teeth of monkeys (*Macaca irus*). *Arch. Oral Biol.* **18**, 669.

Picton D. C. A. and Moss J. P. (1980) The effect on approximal drift of altering the horizontal component of biting force in adult monkeys (*Macaca irus*) *Arch. Oral Biol.* **25**, 45.

Picton D. C. A. and Slater J. M. (1972) The effect on horizontal tooth mobility of experimental trauma to the periodontal membrane in regions of tension or compression in monkeys. *J. Periodont. Res.* **7**, 35.

Poole D. F. G. and Shellis R. P. (1976) Eruptive tooth movements in non-mammalian vertebrates. In: Poole D. F. G. and Stack M. V. (ed), *The Eruption and Occlusion of Teeth*. Proceedings of the 27th Symposium of the Colston Research Society, Bristol, 3–7 April 1975. London, Butterworths, pp. 65–79.

Poole D. F. G. and Stack M. V. (ed) (1976) *The Eruption and Occlusion of Teeth*. Proceedings of the 27th Symposium of the Colston Research Society, Bristol, 3–7 April 1975. London, Butterworths.

Ten Cate A. R. (1969) The mechanism of tooth eruption. In: Melcher A. H. and Bowen W. H. (ed.), *Biology of the Periodontium*. London, Academic, p. 91.

Ten Cate A. R. (1972) Morphological studies of fibrocytes in connective tissue undergoing rapid remodelling. *J. Anat.* **112**, 401.

Ten Cate A. R., Deporter D. A. and Freeman E. (1976) The role of the fibroblasts in the remodelling of periodontal ligament during physiologic tooth movement. *Am. J. Orthod.* **69**, 155.

Thomas N. R. (1967) The properties of collagen in the periodontium of an erupting tooth. In: *The Mechanisms of Tooth Support*. A symposium, Oxford, 6–8 July 1965. Bristol, Wright.

Thomas N. R. (1969) The effect of inhibition of collagen maturation on eruption in rats. *J. Dent. Res.* **44**, 1159.

van Hassel H, J. and McMinn R. G. (1972) Pressure differential favouring tooth eruption in the dog. *J. Dent. Res.* **17**, 183.

Yilmaz R. S., Darling A. I. and Levers B. G. H. (1980) Mesial drift of human teeth assessed from ankylosed deciduous molars. *Arch. Oral Biol.* **25**, 127.

CHAPTER 21

THE DENTO-GINGIVAL JUNCTION

The tooth develops in the bone of jaw and must erupt to assume its functional position. As a result the tooth pierces the oral mucosa and a junction is established between them—a unique circumstance as other similar ectodermal derivatives such as hair follicles, nails or glands are invaginations always with a complete epithelial lining. It could be argued that the junction of oral epithelium to enamel (an epithelial product) represents epithelial continuity, but the fact is that a 'junction' between epithelium and tooth exists and indeed, with age, the nature of the junction changes and is between epithelium and cement—a mesenchymal product covering the root surface. The interruption in epithelial continuity of the lining mucosa of the mouth is, unfortunately, a natural weak point and is the site of onset of most periodontal lesions.

EPITHELIUM

The dento-gingival junction consists of epithelial and connective tissue components. Three anatomically distinct types of epithelium can be distinguished. First, there is the keratinized stratified squamous epithelium of the gingiva which is continuous at the crest of the gingiva with the second type of epithelium, the sulcular or crevicular epithelium. Sulcular epithelium lines the gingival sulcus, faces the tooth and is stratified, squamous and non-keratinized. At the base of the sulcus the crevicular epithelium is continuous with the junctional epithelium. This epithelium has a structure different again from both the gingival and crevicular epithelium and is responsible for the attachment of the gingiva to the tooth. It is characterized by cells having a high rate of cell division, a low nuclear cytoplasmic ratio with significant amounts of rough endoplasmic reticulum in the cytoplasm and with widened spaces between the cells.

The way attachment of this latter epithelium to dental tissue is achieved is understood. Epithelial cells attach to each other by means of a structural entity called the desmosome. A desmosome consists of components contributed by the two cells in contact with each other (*see Fig. 2.3c*). Where a plasma membrane approaches a region of contact its two layers, as seen with the electron microscope, thicken considerably. The cytoplasm on the inner aspect of this thickened part of the plasma membrane is more electron dense and numerous tonofilaments radiate from here into the cell.

This arrangement is repeated in the adjacent cell and a fine electron-dense line can be distinguished in the narrow gap between the two cells. When an epithelial cell, however, is in contact with connective tissue the electron microscope shows that its cell membrane develops only half of this structural unit, the hemi-desmosome. In addition, adjacent to the connective tissue, the cell secretes the lamina lucida and the lamina densa which together form the 'basal lamina'. The mechanism whereby epithelial cells attach to the tooth is thought to be identical to the mechanism whereby such cells attach to connective tissue. Thus the epithelial cells adjacent to the enamel surface possess hemi-desmosomes and are in contact with a basal lamina just as in any other epithelial connective tissue junction (*Fig. 21.1*).

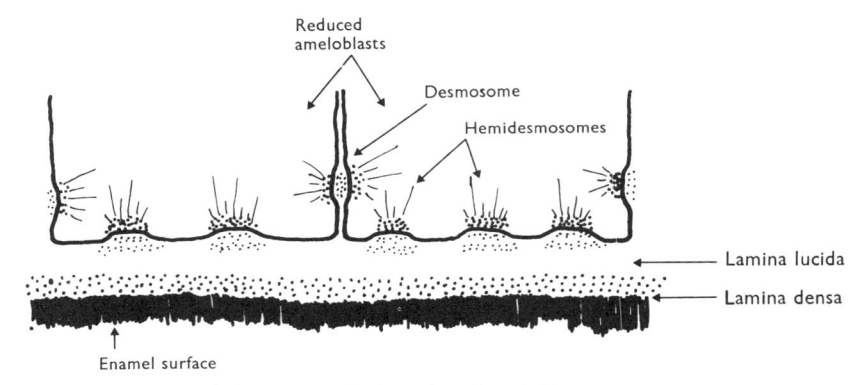

Fig. 21.1. Hemi-desmosomes in the reduced ameloblasts.

CONNECTIVE TISSUE

The connective tissue supporting the epithelium of the dento-gingival junction also shows variation in morphology. The connective tissue supporting the gingival epithelium contains many collagen fibres and fibroblasts with no neutrophils or vesiculated fibroblasts, whereas in the connective tissue adjacent to the sulcular and junctional epithelium there are few collagen fibrils, many neutrophils and vesiculated fibroblasts. It has been observed that these features are similar to, but much less pronounced, than those seen during early gingival inflammation. It would thus appear that even in clinically healthy gingival tissues inflammatory changes are present in connective tissue supporting the epithelium facing the tooth. As inflammation exists in this connective tissue adjacent to the tooth, it is clear that the epithelial seal between the gingiva and the tooth is not adequate for antigens are able to permeate the epithelium and maintain an inflammatory response in the connective tissue.

THE DENTO-GINGIVAL JUNCTION
HOW IS THE ANATOMY OF THE JUNCTION DETERMINED?

The anatomy of the junction is illustrated in *Fig. 21.2* and this configuration raises many interesting questions, including the control of differentiation of three closely juxtaposed epithelia and the reason for the epithelium around the tooth being supported by inflamed connective tissue, whereas elsewhere in the mouth epithelium seems to provide an adequate seal to the ingress of antigens.

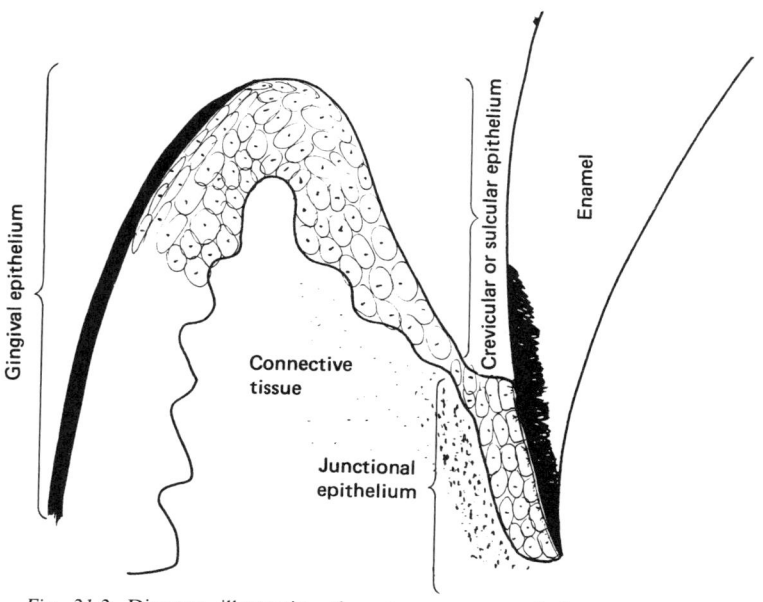

Fig. 21.2. Diagram illustrating the micro-anatomy of the dento-gingival junction. The stippling of the connective tissue indicates inflammation.

Answers to some of these questions may possibly be found in the developmental history of the tooth. Before expounding on this statement two characteristics of epithelium must be described. First, it is well known that there is a dependence between epithelium and the connective tissue which supports it. Some examples of this dependence have been discussed in Chapter 4. Further examples come from simple grafting experiments such as when keratinized epithelium, with its supporting connective tissue, is grafted onto a non-keratinized site (say, to the floor of the vestibular sulcus). The graft remains keratinized. Conversely, if basal epithelial cells from a keratinizing epithelium which are divorced from their connective tissue support are seeded onto a connective tissue site previously supporting non-keratinized epithelium, they form a non-keratinized epithelium.

Second, there are now several reports which indicate that basal epithelial cells respond in a similar way when their local environment is disturbed. These responses include a shift in the cells' metabolic cycle from the citric acid (hexose) cycle to the pentose shunt, lipid synthesis, an increase in cytoplasm and rough endoplasmic reticulum, enlarged extracellular spaces and increased cell division.

Now consider again tooth development. At the beginning of this chapter it was pointed out that the tooth develops within the jaw—divorced from the oral epithelium which gave rise to the enamel or dental organ. This separation is the result of degeneration of the dental lamina which occurs at the bell stage of development. The tooth thus develops separated from the oral epithelium and to function the tooth must erupt and the histological changes which take place to accommodate eruption are as follows.

As the tooth begins to erupt its enamel surface is covered by the reduced enamel epithelium which consists of an outer layer of polygonal epithelial cells, the remnants of the stratum intermedium, stellate reticulum and external dental epithelium and an inner layer of reduced ameloblasts. The ameloblasts at this stage are short columnar cells which have lost their brush border present during enamel maturation (Chapter 22). Instead the cell border adjacent to the enamel is relatively straight and has developed hemi-desmosomes which attach the ameloblast, and therefore the reduced enamel epithelium, firmly to the enamel.

For the tooth to erupt the connective tissue supporting both the reduced enamel epithelium and the oral epithelium must be removed. As this occurs, the cells of the outer layer of the reduced enamel epithelium and the basal cells of the oral epithelium both proliferate forming a mass of epithelial cells over the tooth through which the tooth erupts without ever exposing connective tissue to the external environment (*Fig. 21.3*). This explains why tooth eruption takes place without haemorrhage.

An increased proliferative response is characteristic of any epithelium supported by a connective tissue exhibiting physiological degradation. Another characteristic response is the development of widened spaces between epithelial cells. It is well established that as the reduced enamel epithelium and oral epithelium fuse an acute inflammatory response occurs in the connective tissue around the tooth and the suggestion is that this response is occasioned by the passage of antigens from the oral environment through the widened spaces between the epithelial cells. The important sequel is that the dento-gingival junction then develops in association with a connective tissue which is inflamed and it is not surprising, therefore, that the junctional epithelium exhibits most of the characteristics of epithelial cells supported by a disturbed connective tissue; namely, wide intercellular spaces, high mitotic rate, the presence of increased profiles of rough endoplasmic reticulum and a low nuclear cytoplasmic ratio. The acute inflammation associated with tooth eruption

THE DENTO-GINGIVAL JUNCTION

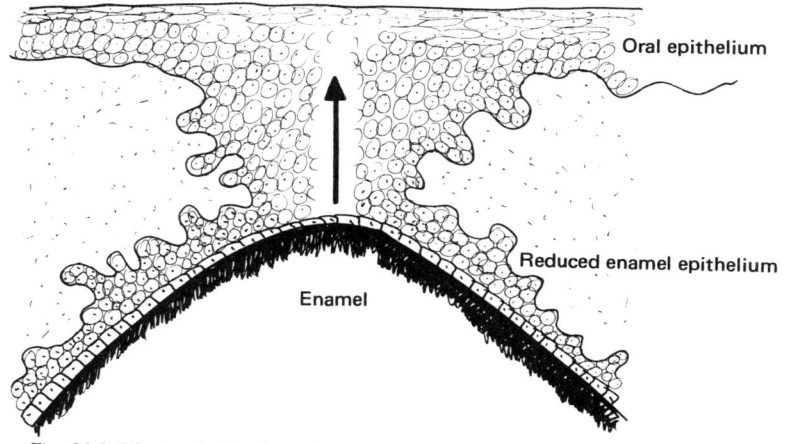

Fig. 21.3. The tooth develops through an epithelial plug developed from an admixture of oral and dental epithelium.

(clinically described as teething) rapidly subsides once the tooth has broken through the oral epithelium. With an epithelial junction at this time exhibiting widened intercellular spaces continued ingress of antigens is possible and a low grade inflammatory state is maintained in the connective tissue around the tooth. Because the junction is developing in association with this inflamed connective tissue, it is possible that this influences, if not determines, the anatomy of the epithelium of the junction.

TESTING THE HYPOTHESIS

This possibility certainly seems to hold for crevicular epithelium and this has been tested in two different ways. If the non-keratinized epithelium of the gingival sulcus and its supporting inflamed connective tissue is grafted to a site away from the tooth, inflammation is lost from the connective tissue and the epithelium keratinizes. Similarly, in experimental animals such as the monkey, when rigid oral hygiene, combined with antibiotic therapy in situ, is practised, inflammation in the connective tissue around the tooth is diminished and keratinization or crevicular epithelium results. Clearly connective tissue plays a role in determining the anatomy of the epithelium lining the crevice.

Whether the inflamed connective tissue also determines the anatomy of the junctional epithelium is a more difficult question to answer. A first examination would seem to indicate that this would be the case. Stereological analysis of junctional epithelium shows its cells to have more cytoplasm, fewer desmosomes, widened intercellular spaces and larger volumes of endoplasmic reticulum—all features of epithelial cells supported by disturbed connective tissue.

If the junctional epithelium were modified by removing inflammation in its supporting connective tissue, the epithelium would likely keratinize. But a keratinized epithelium cannot form an attachment and therefore any attachment would be limited to the deepest and least differentiated cells of the junctional epithelium. Thus it has been suggested that, as the junctional epithelium must adhere to the tooth, an intrinsic degree of permeability must be accepted and in turn an inevitable presence of inflammatory infiltrate in the connective tissue of the gingiva.

It has also been suggested that the differing anatomy of the epithelia associated with the junction is the result of their differing developmental origins. As the tooth erupts, and for some time afterwards, the junction consists of what is called the primary attachment (*Fig. 21.4*). At the cement–enamel junction the enamel surface is covered by the reduced enamel epithelium consisting of clearly recognizable ameloblasts and an outer layer, the remnants of the remainder of the dental organ. Further

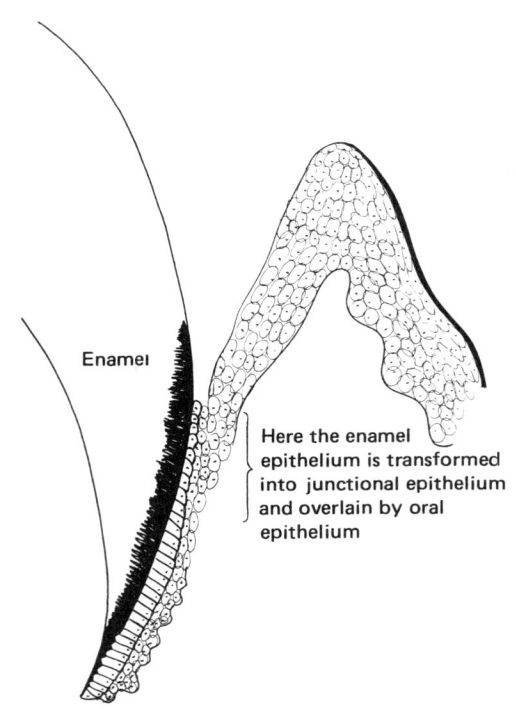

Fig. 21.4. The primary epithelial attachment associated with the newly erupted tooth.

coronally the reduced enamel epithelium is transformed into a squamous epithelium (junctional epithelium) which even more coronally is overlain by a proliferative tongue of epithelium derived from the epithelial cuff. Clearly at this time the junctional epithelium has its origins from the dental epithelium and the transformation to the normal anatomy of the dento-gingival junction is brought about by turnover of the junctional epithelium. However, experiments where the dento-gingival connection is either totally or partially removed and its repair studied reveal that junctional epithelium does not contribute to the re-formation of the junction. Thus, when the junction is totally removed, regeneration of the three distinct epithelial components occurs from cells emanating from oral epithelium. When the oral and sulcular components of the junctional complex are ablated, the remaining junctional epithelium cells form a small nest of epithelial cells in the connective tissue and do not contribute to re-formation of the new junctional epithelium. Junctional epithelium is again derived from basal oral epithelial cells. Thus, junctional epithelium, and therefore dental epithelium, is not necessary to re-form an attachment and, instead, it seems that undifferentiated oral epithelial cells have the capacity to differentiate into the differing epithelia which go to make up the junction. It has been shown that the connective tissue has some role in this differentiation; the question that remains is whether or not the external environment (the tooth surface) has any influence upon epithelial determination.

It is also worth mentioning that previously most workers have assumed that, as sulcular epithelium is not keratinized, this epithelium is permeable and that by changing this tissue to keratinizing epithelium its permeability will be reduced thereby decreasing the potential for periodontal inflammation. It has been pointed out that this assumption may not be valid as there is experimental evidence that uninflamed non-keratinized epithelium is almost as impermeable (or permeable) as keratinized oral epithelium; that epidermal callus is more permeable to water than the stratum corneum of normal skin. Rather than equating permeability with keratinization it is more logical to look at the possible modification of the intercellular substances between epithelial cells. Even so, it must still be recognized that inflammation modifies the property of sulcular epithelium and increases its permeability but perhaps it is more important to recognize that it is the junctional epithelium which offers the pathway of least resistance to those antigens which maintain an inflammatory state in the connective tissue around teeth.

THE COL

Finally, a word about the 'col'. This structure describes the dento-gingival junction interproximally, that is, between the teeth. At first glance the anatomy of the col seems distinctive and for many years it was thought that the reduced enamel epithelium persisted in the col and was therefore a potentially weak covering and the site of onset of periodontal disease. As *Fig. 21.5* explains the epithelium of the col is in fact junctional epithelium and the incidence of gingivitis interdentally is more properly a reflection of the fact that plaque and food debris accumulate interdentally.

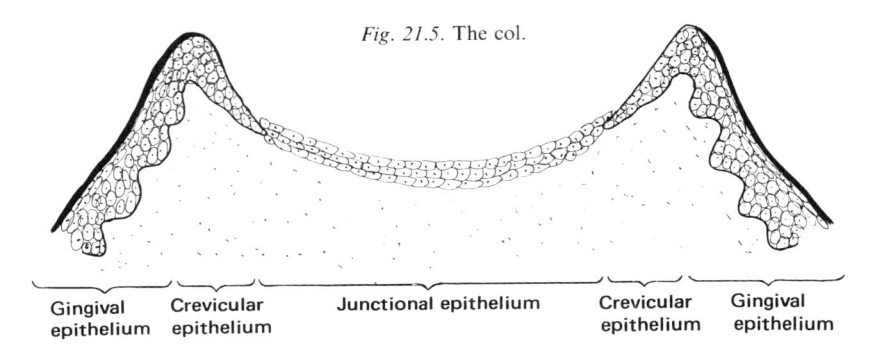

Fig. 21.5. The col.

| Gingival epithelium | Crevicular epithelium | Junctional epithelium | Crevicular epithelium | Gingival epithelium |

REFERENCES AND FURTHER READING

Attstrom R. (1970) Presence of leukocytes in crevices of healthy and chronically inflamed gingivae. *J. Periodont. Res.* **5**, 42.

Attstrom R. and Egelberg J. (1970) Emigration of blood neutrophils and monocytes into the gingival crevices. *J. Periodont. Res.* **5**, 48.

Brill N. and Bjorn H. (1959) Passage of tissue fluid into human gingival pockets. *Acta Odont. Scand.* **17**, 11.

Brill N. and Krasse B. (1958) The passage of tissue fluid into the clinically healthy gingival pocket. *Acta Odont. Scand.* **16**, 233.

Caffesse R. G., Karring T. and Nasjleti C. E. (1977) Keratinizing potential of sulcular epithelium. *J. Periodont.* **48**, 140.

Caffesse R. G., Kornman K. S. and Nasjleti C. E. (1980) The effect of intensive antibacterial therapy on the sulcular environment in monkeys. Part II. Inflammation, mitotic activity and keratinization of the sulcular epithelium. *J. Periodont.* **51**, 155.

Caffesse R. G., Nasjleti C. E. and Castelli W. A. (1979) The role of sulcular environment in controlling epithelial keratinization. *J. Periodont.* **50**, 6.

Engler W. O., Ramfjord S. P. and Hiniker J. J. (1965) Development of epithelial attachment and gingival sulcus in rhesus monkeys. *J. Periodont.* **36**, 44.

Frank R., Fiore-Donno G., Cimasoni G. et al. (1974) Ultrastructural study of epithelial and connective gingival reattachment in man. *J. Periodont.* **45**, 626.

Garant P. R. and Mulvihill J. E. (1971) The ultrastructure of clinically normal sulcular tissues in the beagle dog. *J. Periodont. Res.* **6**, 252.

Gargiulo A. W., Wentz F. M. and Orban B. (1961) Dimensions and relations of the dentogingival junction in humans. *J. Periodont.* **32**, 261.

Gavin J. B. (1968) The ultrastructure of the crevicular epithelium of cat gingiva. *Am. J. Anat.* **123**, 283.

Geisenheimer J. and Han S. S. (1971) A quantitative electron microscopic study of desmosomes and hemidesmosomes in human crevicular epithelium. *J. Periodont.* **42**, 396.

Gelfand H. B., Ten Cate A. R. and Freeman E. (1978) The keratinization potential of crevicular epithelium: an experimental study. *J. Periodont.* **49**, 113.

Glavind L. and Zander H. A. (1970) Dynamics of dental epithelium during tooth eruption. *J. Dent. Res.* **49**, 549.

Innes P. B. (1970) An electron microscopic study of the regeneration of gingival epithelium following gingivectomy in the dog. *J. Periodont. Res.* **5**, 196.

Innes P. B. (1971) The differentiation of cat crevicular epithelium in diffusion chambers *in vivo*. *Anat. Rec.* **169**, 345.

Ito H., Enomoto S. and Kobayashi K. (1967a) Electron microscopic study of the human epithelial attachment. *Bull. Tokyo Med. Dent. Univ.* **14**, 267.

Ito H., Enomoto S. and Kobayashi K. (1967b) Electron microscopic study of the human epithelial attachment. *Bull. Tokyo Med. Dent. Univ.* **14**, 267.

Karring T., Lang N. P. and Loe H. (1975) The role of gingival tissue in determining epithelial differentiation. *J. Periodont. Res.* **10**, 1.

Kornman K. S., Caffesse R. G. and Nasjleti C. E. (1980) The effect of intensive antibacterial therapy on the sulcular environment in monkeys. Part I. Changes in the bacteriology of the gingival sulcus. *J. Periodont.* **51**, 34.

Listgarten M. A. (1966a) Phase-contrast and electron microscopic study of the junction between reduced enamel epithelium and enamel in unerupted human teeth. *Arch. Oral Biol.* **11**, 999.

Listgarten M. A. (1966b) Electron microscopic study of the dento-gingival junction of man. *Am. J. Anat.* **119**, 147.

Listgarten M. A. (1967) Electron microscopic features of the newly formed epithelial attachment after gingival surgery. *J. Periodont. Res.* **2**, 46.

Listgarten M. A. (1970) Changing concepts about the dento-epithelial junction. *J. Can. Dent. Assoc.* **36**, 70.

Listgarten M. A. (1972a) Ultrastructure of the dento-gingival junction after gingivectomy. *J. Periodont. Res.* **7**, 151.

Listgarten M. A. (1972b) Normal development, structure, physiology and repair of gingival epithelium. In: *Gingival Epithelium. Oral Science Reviews*. Vol. 1. Copenhagen, Munksgaard, p. 3.

McHugh W. D. (1961) The development of the gingival epithelium in the monkey. *Dent. Practnr Dent. Rec.* **11**, 314.

McHugh W. D. (1971) The interdental gingivae. *J. Periodont. Res.* **6**, 227.

McHugh W. D. and Zander H. A. (1965) Cell division in the periodontium of developing and erupted teeth. *Dent. Practnr Dent. Rec.* **15**, 451.

Magnusson B. (1968) Tissue changes during molar tooth eruption. *Trans. R. Sch. Dent. Stockholm, Umea.* **13**, 1.

Magnusson B. (1969) Mucosal changes at erupting molars in germ-free rats. *J. Periodont. Res.* **4**, 181.

Provenza D. V. and Sisca R. F. (1970) Fine structure features of monkey (*Macaca mulata*) reduced enamel epithelium. *J. Periodont.* **41**, 313.

Schroeder H. E. (1969) Ultrastructure of the junctional epithelium of the human gingiva. *Helv. Odont. Acta* **13**, 65.

Schroeder H. E. and Listgarten M. A. (1971) Fine structure of the developing epithelial attachment of human teeth. In: Wolsky A., (ed.), *Monographs in Developmental Biology*, vol. 2. Basel, Karger.

Schroeder H. E. and Munzel-Pedrazzoli S. (1970) Morphometric analysis comparing junctional and oral epithelium of normal human gingiva. *Helv. Odont. Acta* **14**, 53.

Skougaard M. and Beagrie G. S. (1962) The renewal of gingival epithelium in marmosets (*Calithrix jacchus*) as determined through autoradiography with thymidine-H. *Acta Odont. Scand.* **20**, 467.

Ten Cate A. R. (1971) Physiological resorption of connective tissue associated with tooth eruption. *J. Periodont. Res.* **6**, 168.

Ten Cate A. R. (1975) The dento-gingival junction. An interpretation of the literature. *J. Periodont.* **46**, 475.

CHAPTER 22

THE FINAL INVESTMENTS OF THE CROWN OF THE TOOTH

In the past century the two-layered appearance of a membrane which covers newly erupted teeth was described (*Fig. 22.1a, b*). The outer layer of this membrane is cellular and probably consists entirely of the remnants of the enamel organ which covered the fully developed enamel. For obvious reasons this cellular layer is called the 'reduced enamel epithelium'. The inner layer, about whose presence there has been disagreement, is about 1 μm thick, is not always seen and has a structureless refractile appearance. It was called the 'primary enamel cuticle'. The two layers, cellular and acellular, are known together as 'Nasmyth's membrane'.

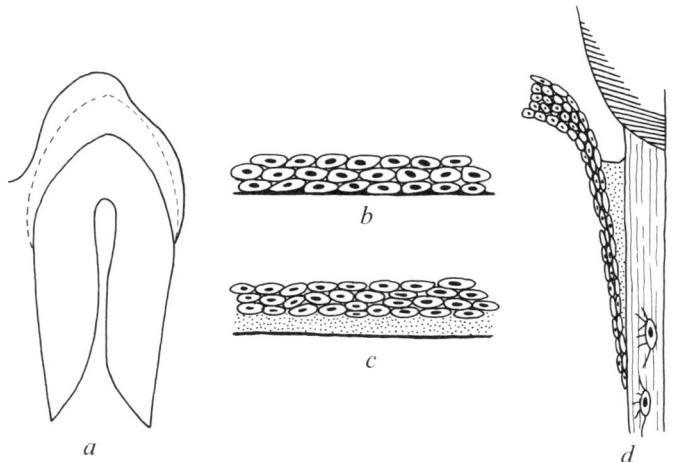

Fig. 22.1. When a recently erupted tooth is dissolved in acid a membrane floats from the surface of the dissolved enamel (Nasmyth's membrane, *a*). This consists of the reduced enamel epithelium and possibly a thin inner structureless layer, the primary enamel cuticle (*b*). Sometimes a much thicker structureless layer, with different staining properties, intervenes between the two layers (secondary enamel cuticle, stippled in *c*), although the primary cuticle indicated in this diagram is usually not seen. A secondary enamel cuticle (stippled in *d*) may also separate the cement from the epithelial attachment.

DEVELOPMENT OF NASMYTH'S MEMBRANE

The reduced enamel epithelium contains two cell types. An inner layer of 'reduced ameloblasts' can be recognized until about the time at which the tooth erupts (*Fig. 22.2a–c*). Between the end of amelogenesis and the eruption of the tooth (a period of about 3 years for the first permanent molar) these cells 'degenerate' from columnar, to cuboidal, to squamous. They adhere to the surface of the enamel by means of a basal lamina and hemi-desmosomes (*Fig. 22.2d–e*). The remainder of the cells of the enamel organ (stratum intermedium, external dental epithelium and perhaps some stellate reticulum) which, it will be recalled, are already squamous at the end of amelogenesis, become the outer layer of reduced enamel epithelium and are capable of dividing. It is not known what happens in the next year or two but by the time the tooth begins to move towards the oral cavity the enamel is covered by an actively proliferating reduced enamel epithelium which has generated a basal lamina together with the associated hemi-desmosomes (Chapter 21).

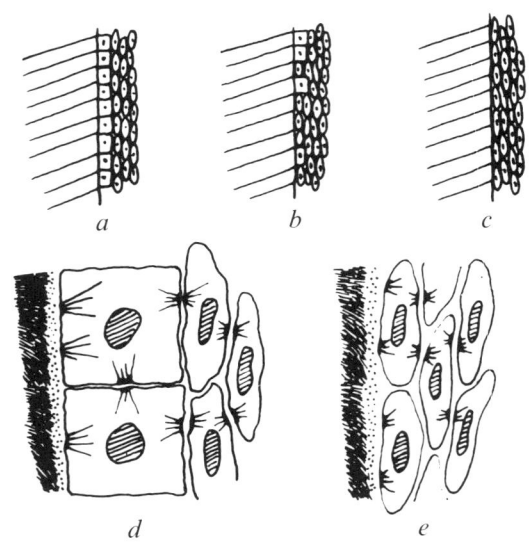

Fig. 22.2. The replacement (or conversion) of reduced ameloblasts by more squamous cells (*a–c*). *d* and *e* are high-power views of *a* and *c*.

As the tooth erupts, proliferating cells of the reduced enamel epithelium mingle with proliferating cells of the oral epithelium to become the first 'junctional epithelium', i.e. that epithelium which forms a junction between enamel and what is obviously oral epithelium (*see Fig. 21.3*). Later that part of the tooth beyond the junctional epithelium, and well into the oral cavity, may still retain a few adherent cells (? reduced ameloblasts, or cells from the proliferating layer of the reduced enamel epithelium, or perhaps cells from junctional epithelium) (*Fig. 22.3b*).

THE FINAL INVESTMENTS OF THE CROWN

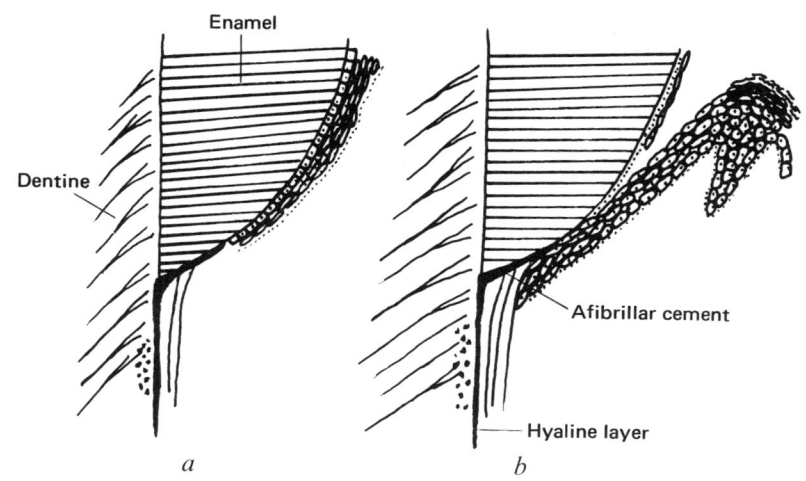

Fig. 22.3. a, Following crown formation and prior to tooth eruption, the reduced enamel epithelium 'contracts' away from the cervical margin of the tooth exposing enamel to the tooth follicle. Afibrillar cement (black) is laid down. Later, acellular cement is deposited on this cement. *b,* The cervical enamel of an erupted tooth may be covered by a cuticle of greatly thickened basement lamina material (dotted line). Some cells from the junctional epithelium may adhere to this cuticle. In this diagram afibrillar cement is shown continuous with the hyaline layer of dentine.

POSSIBLE ORIGIN OF DENTAL CUTICLES

The term 'cuticle' is used to describe any layer which lies on the surface of the erupted or unerupted enamel or on the cement and is secreted by adjacent cells. The term 'pellicle' describes layers on the erupted tooth surface which are derived from either the saliva or adherent bacteria.

There are several possible sources of cuticle amongst which are ameloblasts, reduced enamel epithelium (REE), follicular cells that have penetrated the REE, and junctional epithelium. At one time or another all these can lie on the enamel surface.

Ameloblasts

It was originally proposed that the final secretions of the ameloblast may remain unmineralized, or be only partially mineralized, and continuous with the enamel matrix between crystals. The structureless layer would be a cuticle (in this case the primary cuticle).

Reduced Enamel Epithelium

The inner surface of the REE is attached to the enamel by a basal lamina and hemi-desmosomes. This basal lamina satisfies the definition of a cuticle.

Follicular Cells

The enamel of the long-crowned teeth of hypsodont mammals is covered by cement. Before the tooth erupts the enamel organ breaks down and cement is deposited on the exposed enamel. Small regions of cement can often be seen on the enamel of human teeth and could be termed cuticular in this situation.

Junctional Epithelium

This is attached to the surface of the erupted tooth by a basal lamina and hemi-desmosomes. Such a basal lamina first lies on enamel but is later secreted on the cement when the epithelial attachment has migrated on to the root. In both situations the basal lamina is a cuticle.

One final structure has been described which could be confused with a cuticle as defined here. It is suggested (Hodson, 1966a) following a slight injury that blood could leak through REE or junctional epithelium and come to lie on the surface of the tooth (enamel or cement). Much of the blood would be absorbed back through the epithelium but large molecular weight materials such as globin would remain and condense to form a layer resembling a cuticle.

STRUCTURE OF CUTICLES

Dental cuticles are between 30 nm and 5 µm thick, and are largely structureless. A recent study (Newman, 1980) concluded that all cuticles are continuous with organic matter in the surface enamel. This does not mean that they all consist of enamel matrix, merely that they lack structure and have similar densities when viewed by electron microscopy.

Both thin and thick cuticles consist of protein possibly together with proteoglycan. From the above it seems that most cuticles may originate as basal lamina from the epithelia which cover teeth. In other situations basal laminae are about 50 nm wide and are probably subject to continuous turnover; secretion by epithelium and absorption by epithelium or adjacent mesoderm. On the surface of the tooth, the basal lamina is 'outside' the body and may not be subject to the same turnover. Depending on its condition the adjacent epithelium may maintain a narrow cuticle either by secretion and absorption or by failing to produce more basal lamina material. Alternatively, the epithelium may fail to absorb lamina but continue secreting it with the result that a thick cuticle is built. No explanation for these differences has been offered.

Cement on the enamel surface, in common with most root cement, contains collagen fibres. However, a type of mineralized tissue without collagen fibres has been described and given the name 'afibrillar cement'. This could be equivalent to a thin layer of material secreted by root sheath cells onto the surface of the root dentine (in rat and dog) and later mineralized by cementoblasts. Afibrillar cement is uncommon and is located at the neck of the tooth.

FUNCTION OF CUTICLES

A basal lamina is always present between epithelia and mesoderm and together with hemi-desmosomes in the epithelia may be required to attach the layers. Epithelial cells grown in culture attach to glass by means of the same mechanism. It therefore seems that normal healthy junctional epithelium needs to produce a basal lamina, perhaps 50 nm thick, to become attached to the enamel or cement surface. What of the other types of cuticle, and the (possible?) basal lamina material which may be 100 times thicker? Little is known, not even whether they are normal or pathological.

PELLICLES

Organic layers attached to the tooth surface may be dried saliva, food debris, bacteria and bacterial products. Such pellicles may become mineralized to produce a hard, adherent 'calculus'.

Pellicles do not really concern us here. They are, however, of great importance in the onset of both caries and periodontal disease.

REFERENCES AND FURTHER READING

Dawes C., Jenkins G. N. and Tonge C. H. (1963) The nomenclature of the integuments of the enamel surface of teeth. *Br. Dent. J.* **115**, 65.

Hodson J. J. (1966a) The distribution, structure, origin and nature of the dental cuticle of Gottlieb, Part I and Part II. *J. Am. Soc. Periodont.* **5**, 237, 295.

Hodson J. J. (1966b) Electron microscopic study of the gingivo-dental junction of man. *Am. J. Anat.* **119**, 147.

Melcher A. H. and Zarb G. A. (ed.) (1972) *Gingival Epithelium. Oral Sciences Reviews*, vol. 1. Copenhagen, Munskgaard.

Newman H. N. (1980) Ultrastructural observations on the human pre-eruptive enamel cuticle. *Arch. Oral Biol.* **25**, 49.

Provenze D. V. and Sisca R. F. (1970) Fine structure features of monkey (*Macaca mulatta*) reduced enamel epithelium. *J. Periodont.* **4**, 313.

For further references, *see* Chapter 21.

CHAPTER 23

AGE CHANGES IN THE DENTAL TISSUES

In animal wildlife teeth are such important structures that the loss of the dentition marks the end of an animal's life span. Although this is not true of modern man the teeth exhibit senescent phenomena which are important. Perhaps the most important age changes are the wear of enamel (because it cannot be replaced) and the apical retreat of the epithelial attachment (which must eventually lead to the loss of the tooth).

ENAMEL

Enamel is a relatively inert tissue because it has no cellular component. However, certain age changes take place in response to attrition and to physico-chemical changes in structure.

The most conspicuous age change associated with enamel is its loss due to wear. This loss is extremely variable depending on the diet of the individual, the nature of the occlusion and the composition of the enamel. Occlusal wear due to attrition (tooth/tooth contact) and abrasion (tooth/food/tooth contact) is obvious. It has been shown to improve the efficiency of human teeth (Dahlberg, 1942); the greater the area of occlusal contact the more efficiently the dentition processes food (Osborn and Lumsden, 1978). Attrition also occurs at the contact points between teeth due to the different movements of adjacent teeth during mastication, and the extent of this wear can be considerable. It has been estimated that by the age of 40 as much as 1 cm can be lost from the overall circumferential length of the arch in the average complete dentition (Black, 1924). Finally, the buccal and lingual surfaces of enamel are worn, obliterating the perikymata and other surface markings.

The use of dyes and radioactive isotopes has shown conclusively that enamel is slightly permeable, and that this permeability decreases with age. It seems that ions are exchanged between the surface enamel and saliva. It is usually thought that fluoride is most beneficial in preventing caries if it can be incorporated into developing enamel.

Several recent studies, however, suggest that the benefits of a fluoridated water supply are not so much due to the incorporation of fluorine into developing teeth as due to the continual washing of the tooth surfaces every time water is drunk. This indicates the importance of ionic exchange at the tooth surface.

Teeth darken with age. Either the enamel picks up stains or, because the enamel is thinner due to wear, the underlying yellowish dentine is seen more clearly. Hair-line cracks running vertically through the enamel are often seen in older teeth. One suggestion is that age changes in the dentine lead to its contraction. The poorly supported enamel now cracks and organic material from saliva enters the crack and subsequently becomes stained.

There is little evidence for any age change in the organic matrix of enamel. This is not surprising in view of the very limited permeability of the tissue. In summary, all the age changes described above are physico-chemical.

DENTINE

Age changes in the dentine are more marked because, unlike enamel, this tissue is vital. The formation of dentine continues throughout life but at a diminishing rate, so that the volume of the pulp chamber progressively diminishes by the development of physiological (or regular) secondary dentine. This is not necessarily a response to occlusal wear since by age 30 as much secondary dentine has formed in unerupted molars as in equivalent erupted teeth. Furthermore, the formation of this dentine begins on the side walls of incisors rather than under the incisal tips.

Although not easy to distinguish by conventional microscopy, a marked difference has been shown between the matrix of physiological secondary dentine and the far more rapidly formed primary dentine. Also, contrary to previous descriptions, it has now been claimed that this secondary dentine has considerably fewer tubules than primary dentine.

A third form of dentine may be deposited in response to advancing attrition and dental disease. This is pathological (or irregular) secondary dentine in which a severely reduced number of tubules pursue a haphazard course. The reduced number of tubules is due to the death of many odontoblasts and the haphazard course, presumably, to the absence of restraints from adjacent odontoblasts. The formation of pathological secondary dentine is by no means an inevitable response to wear and disease. In one study only about a half of the carious teeth had responded in this way. Pathological secondary dentine has what would seem to be the advantageous property of being much less permeable than primary and physiological secondary dentines.

The above two age changes involve additions of secondary dentine to the primary dentine. Two further age changes, transparent dentine and dead tracts, involve alterations to existing dentine. In transparent (sclerotic) dentine the tubules are progressively occluded, by deposition within their lumina of mineral salts, so that the now mineralized tubules have the same refractive index as inter-tubular dentine. It is thought that the tubules become filled with peri-tubular dentine. Although translucent dentine can develop anywhere in the dentine, it is consistently found in the root region after middle age. Teeth containing translucent dentine appear to be more brittle than other teeth making them more liable to fracture during extraction.

In the formation of a dead tract the odontoblast processes degenerate leaving empty tubules. Such tubules are, however, sealed off at their pulpal end by the deposition of pathological (irregular) secondary dentine. When viewed in transmitted light, dead tracts appear more opaque than normal dentine due to the presence of air in the empty tubules. Although translucent dentine and dead tracts frequently form in response to attrition or dental disease, there is ample evidence that both changes can be independent of peripheral injuries, and they must consequently be regarded as progressive age changes within dentine.

In contrast to the age changes in enamel, those in dentine are all mediated by cells.

CEMENT

Cement is deposited intermittently throughout life around the roots of teeth and there is a loose correlation between the thickness of cement and age. This relationship is a linear one, but the thickness of cement is too readily influenced by the functional stresses applied to the tooth and by periodontal disease to provide a wholly reliable indication of dental age.

PULP

With the initial completion of the apex of the root the dental pulp can be considered to have attained maturity. The pulp has been shown to be similar in composition, organization and histo-chemical reactivity to other connective tissues, and it bears the same relationship to dentine as bone marrow to mineralized bone. Functionally, pulp and dentine should be regarded as the two parts of one tissue and in consequence some of the age changes of dentine are also age changes of the pulp.

The young pulp contains many fibroblasts, young collagen fibres and relatively few mature collagen fibres, all disposed in a fluid ground substance. With advancing age, mature collagen fibres increase in number, cellular elements decrease and the ground substance becomes less aqueous. These changes may be the result of a diminishing blood supply to the pulp consequent upon vascular strangulation by narrowing of the apical canal and upon progressive arteriosclerosis which has been shown to begin in pulpal vessels at about age 40. The perineurium of pulpal nerves becomes mineralized with advancing years and this eventually leads to the obliteration of nerves (? due to diminished vascularity) with the result that the pulp becomes increasingly insensitive.

Radiographs often reveal the presence of mineralized nodules within the pulp cavity of the tooth. Under the light microscope these 'pulp stones' can have one or two appearances. Either the irregularly mineralized nodules may contain a few randomly arranged tubules or they may have the appearance of a relatively acellular bone. The first type is called a true pulp stone (because it contains 'dentinal tubules'), the second a false pulp stone. With the progressive deposition of dentine on the walls of the pulp cavity these stones may finally become embedded on the encroaching pulpal surface of the dentine. Another variety of ectopic mineralization is referred to as 'diffuse calcification of the pulp'. In this case irregular strands (rather than discrete nodules) of poorly mineralized tissue are found distributed throughout the pulp. The origin of pulp stones is unknown. Perhaps, following a minute pulpal haemorrhage, extravasated blood cells form a focus for the development of fibrous tissue which subsequently becomes mineralized. Layers of mineralized tissue are now deposited around this focus to form the discrete mineralized nodule. But this cannot explain the presence of 'dentinal tubules' in a pulp stone. It will be recalled that odontoblasts are only differentiated under the influence of the internal dental epithelium or Hertwig's root sheath and neither of these is present in the pulp. Diffuse calcification of the pulp is probably produced in response to the decreased vascularity of an ageing pulp but the mechanism by which it is produced is not known.

PERIODONTAL LIGAMENT

The periodontal ligament forms the attachment between tooth and bone and the life span of the tooth depends upon its integrity. Little is known of the quantitative and qualitative changes occurring with age within the ligament itself except that it may become narrower. This change is probably related to the forces applied to teeth. The more load a tooth bears, the wider is its ligament. Older people have a less powerful bite with the result that the teeth are less stressed and their ligaments become narrower. Far more attention has been paid to the apical downgrowth of the epithelial attachment with age. Two opinions have been expressed in attempts to explain the cause of the retreat of the attachment. Some consider it is a direct response to inflammatory change in the periodontal ligament, and it is true that in sections of this region some evidence of inflammatory cell infiltration can always be found. An alternative interpretation is that the retreat of the attachment is a physiological process termed 'passive eruption'. In other animals, where gingival disease is not as widespread as in man, slow gingival recession proceeds as an apparently normal age change and this fact has been used as an argument against the belief that inflammatory change is the causative factor.

The problem of passive eruption, which J. H. Scott called 'dental striptease', has been deepened by Ainamo and Talari (1975). He measured the distance of the mucogingival junction of lower teeth from the lower border of the mandible in young and old people and showed there was little or no difference between the age groups. He produced equivalent results for upper teeth using the palate as a marker. Assuming, reasonably, little or no remodelling of the bony landmarks it would have been expected that passive eruption would lower the mucogingival junctions on lower teeth bringing them closer to the lower border of the mandible. The observations are difficult to explain because they seem to suggest, contrary to all clinical impressions, that the gingival attachment does not move and that passive eruption does not exist.

ORAL MUCOSA

Clinical observations give the impression that the oral mucosa in the aged is thinner, dryer and more fragile. What evidence there is suggests that there is diminution in keratinization with age, but this has been obtained from studies involving cytological smears which at best are capricious.

TEETH AS INDICATORS OF AGE

Studies of teeth have proved exceptionally useful in determining the age of mutilated or otherwise unrecognizable bodies. It is obvious that up to the age of 20 the developing and erupting teeth provide an accurate estimate of an individual's age. However, even beyond this time teeth frequently provide very good estimates of age. Longitudinal ground sections of a single tooth or several teeth are prepared. The following five features are studied: attrition, secondary dentine, translucent dentine, the position of the epithelial attachment and the thickness of the cement. Each of these features is given a score from 0 to 3. Zero represents the condition expected in a perfect young tooth whereas 3 represents an extremely advanced stage of, for instance, spread of translucent dentine, attrition or cement thickness. The five scores are added together to give a final figure. Thus a single tooth may score attrition 2, secondary dentine 1, translucent dentine 3, epithelial attachment 1, cement 2. The total is 9. By referring to published tables a good estimate of the age of a person having teeth with a score of 9 can be obtained.

REFERENCES AND FURTHER READING

Ainamo J. and Talari A. (1975) Eruptive movements of teeth in human adults. In: Poole D. F. G. and Stack M. V. (ed.), *The Eruption and Occlusion of Teeth*. London, Butterworths.

Bernick S. (1967) Age changes in the blood supply to human teeth. *J. Dent. Res.* **46**, 544.

Black G. V. (1924) In: *Operative Dentistry*, 6th ed., vol. 1. London, Kimpton, p. 223.

Dahlberg B. (1942) The masticatory effect. *Acta Med. Scand.* Suppl. 139.

Gustafson G. (1950) Age determinations of teeth. *J. Am. Dent. Assoc.* **41**, 45.

Jenkins G. N. (1966) *The Physiology of the Mouth*, 3rd ed. Oxford, Blackwell, pp. 157, 241.

Miles A. E. W. (1963) The dentition in the assessment of individual age in skeletal material In: Brothwell D. R. (ed.), *Dental Anthropology*. Oxford, Pergamon.

Miles A. E. W. (1976) Age changes in dental tissues. In: Cohen B. and Kramer I. R. H. (ed.), *Scientific Foundation of Dentistry*. London, Heinemann.

Osborn J. W. and Lumsden A. S. (1978) An alternative to thegosis and a re-examination of the ways in which mammalian molars work. *N. Jb. Geol. Palaeont.* **156**, 371.

Phillipas G. G. and Applebaum E. (1966) Age factor in secondary dentine formation. *J. Dent. Res.* **45**, 778.

Zander H. A. and Hürzeleger B. (1958) Continuous cementum apposition. *J. Dent. Res.* **37**, 1035.

INDEX

Acetylcholinesterase, dentine content of, 112–13
Acid phosphatase, in ameloblast, 125
  location in sections, 2, (*Fig. 1.1*) 3
Adenosine triphosphate production, 21
Adhesive zones, 16
Age changes in dental tissues, 198–202
Alkaline phosphatase, activity in odontoblasts, 94
  role in mineralization, 77, 80–81, (*Fig. 10.5*) 82, 118, 125
Alveolar bone *see under* Bone
Ameloblasts, as cuticle source, 195
  contents of, 122–3
  differentiation, 119–20, (*Fig. 15.4*) 122
  histology, 121
  reduced, 193–4
  relationship to prisms, 126–35, 138
Amelogenesis, 87–88, 118–35
Amelogenin, 122–3
Amino-acids, analysis of, 8–9
  in collagen, 69
  in enamel, (*Fig. 15.6*) 124
Aminopeptidase in enamel, 125
Apatite crystals, 78, (*Figs. 10.3–4*) 79–80
Apical foramen, 156, (*Fig. 18.1*) 157
Autoradiography techniques, 6–7
Azo-dye staining method, 2, (*Fig. 1.1*) 3

Basement membrane, 23–24
Bell stage of tooth development, 41–42, 47, 118
Biochemical analysis of tissues, 8–9
Blood supply to teeth, 63–67, 165–6, 174, 200
Bone, 89–93
  alveolar, 27, 164
    blood supply to, (*Fig. 8.3*) 66, 67
  cancellous, 90–91
  compact, 90–91
  crypts, 39
  embryonic, (*Fig. 11.1*) 89
  formation, 81–84, 89–92
  grafts, 163
  interstitial, 91
  remodelling, 92–93, 164, 172–3, 177

cAMP role in tooth development, 51
cGMP role in tooth development, 51
Calcium, mineralization pathway of, 98
  mitochondrial storage of, 77, 99
  radioactive marker, 7
Calcium hydroxyapatite, 75, 120
Calcium triphosphate, 75
Calculus, 197
Canines
  clone, 44
  growth of deciduous, 57, (*Fig. 7.2*) 58
  morphology, 53–54
Cap stage of tooth development, 40–41
Cell
  attachments, (*Fig. 2.3*) 17
  condensations, 39
  lineage, 30–31
  nucleus, 18
  pearls, 42
  proliferation, 173
  structure, 12–24
Cement, afibrillar, 150–1, (*Fig. 22.3*) 195, 197
  age changes in, 200
  cellular, 153–4
  classification, 150
  extrinsic fibre, 151–2
  intermediate, 153
  intrinsic fibre, 152
  mixed fibre, 152
  on enamel, 196, 197
  structure, 153–5
Cementoblasts, 151–2
Cementocytes, 153–4
Cementogenesis, 84–85, 150–5
Cementoid, 150, 155
Cervical loop, (*Fig. 3.1*) 25, 26, 159
Chromatographic analysis of protein, 8–9
Clones, dental, 38, 43–44, 54
Col, 189–90
Collagen, 69–74
  degradation, 71–74
  dentine content of, 8, 94–95, 104–5
  effects on tooth movement, 176
  effects on tooth shape, 50–51
  fibres, anchoring tooth, 27
    extrinsic, 152
    periodontal ligament relationship to, 164
  fibrils, 70–71

INDEX

Collagen, fibrils (cont.)
  mineral deposition associated with, (Fig. 10.4) 80, 81
  glycine content of, 8
  molecule, 69–70
  synthesis, 70, 167
  turnover in periodontal ligament, 6–7, 72, 164, 167
  types, 23, 69–70
  type IV in tooth germs, 7–8
Collagenase, 72
Connective tissue, 184, 186–9
Crown, anatomical, 26
  clinical, 26
  development, 41, 49
  final investments of, 193–7
  measurement of, 56
    height, (Fig. 7.4) 60
  relationship to root pattern, 160
Cushion hammock ligament, 173
Cusp, distances between, 56–57
  formation, 48–49, 51–54
  pressure on, 115
  relationship to roots, 160
Cuticles, dental, 195–7
Cytodifferentiation, 46, 47

Dentine, 26
  age changes in, 199–200
  caps, staining and measurement of, 56
  circumpulpal, 95, 96, (Fig. 12.3), 97, 104–5
  collagen in, 8, 94–96, 104–5
  dead tracks, 200
  features of, (Fig. 13.1) 106
  fluid movements in, 113–14, 116
  formation, 48, 85–86, 94–101
  forming blood barrier, 64–65
  hyaline, 150–1
  interglobular, 105
  mantle, 95, 96 (Fig. 12.3) 97, 104
  nerve fibres in, 10, 109–12
  peritubular, 10, 99–100, 105
  primary, 104, 199
  pulp complex, 104–8
  repair, 108
  sclerotic, 105
  secondary, 104, 199
  sensitivity of, 109–16
  tertiary, 104
  transparent, 199–200
  tubules, light microscopy of, 3
    shape of, 100 (Figs. 12.6–7) 101

Dentine (cont.)
  vaso-, 116
Dento-gingival junction, 183–90
Desmosomes, 16, 121, 183–4
Diastema in animals, 37
DNA, 18

Ectomesenchyme, role in tooth formation and induction, 28–33, 39, 50
Electron microscopy, 4–6
Embryo, bone formation in, (Fig. 11.1) 89
  development of head in, (Fig. 5.1) 35
Enamel, 27
  age changes in, 198–9
  calcium uptake in, 7
  caps, staining and measurement of, 56
  cement on, 196, 197
  cord, 41, 42
  cuticle, primary, 193
  deposition rate of, 60
  formation, 87–88, 118–35
  histology, 120–2
  knot, (Fig. 5.2e) 36, 41
  lamellae, 146–8
  light microscopy of, 3
  loss, 198
  matrix, 120, 122–3
  maturation, 124–6
  navel, 42
  organ, folding of, 47–48
  porosity, 144
  reduced epithelium, 193–4, (Fig. 22.3) 195, 196
  root, 26, 160
  septum, 42
  spindles, 146–8
  structure, 137–48
  thickness variations of, 47
  tubules, 147–8
  tufts, 146–8
Enamelin, 123
Endoplasmic reticulum, 20, 121
Eosin staining, 2
Epithelial attachment, blood supply to, 67
Epithelial cell rests of Malassez, 158–9, 164
Epithelium, blood supply to, 64–65
  crevicular, 183
  dental, 26, 27, 189
    development, 35–37, 41
    effects on tooth shape, 50
    growth, 57, 61, 94, 121
    height measurement of, 60

INDEX

Epithelium, blood supply to, dental (*cont.*)
   internal, 47–48, 119
   mesenchymal interactions with, 31–32
   gingival, 183
   grafts, 185–6, 187
   junctional, 183, 187–9, 194, 196
Exocytosis, 15

Fibrillogenesis, 70–71
Fibroblasts, 72–74, 165, 177
Fluid movements in teeth, 113–14, 116, 166, 173–4
Follicle, dental, 161–3
Follicular cells, 196

Gingiva, blood supply to, (*Fig. 8.3*) 66, 67
   fibres, 166
   inflammatory changes in, 184
   recession, 201–2
Gingival margin, 26
Glycine in dentinal collagen, 8
Glycosaminoglycan secretion, 40–41
Golgi apparatus, 20
   material, 121
Gomphosis, 163
Granular layer of Tomes, 26, 107–8
Gubernacular canal, 39
   cord, 39

Haematoxylin staining, 2
Hard tissue *see under* Tissue
Hemi-desmosomes, (*Fig. 21.1*) 184
Hertwig's root sheath, 150, 156–60, 164
Histochemical staining techniques, 2
Histological marker techniques, 6–8
Hunter–Schreger bands, 140, 145
Hypercementosis, 154–5

Immunological marker techniques, 7–8
Incisor
   clone, 43–44
   eruptive movement, 174–5
   growth of deciduous, 57, (*Fig. 7.2*) 58
   morphology, 46, 53–54
Inflammatory effects, 184, (*Fig. 21.2*) 185, 186–7, 201

Intermediate plexus, 167
Investing layer, (*Fig. 19.1*) 161

Jaw growth, 177
Junctional complex, 16
Junctions, gap, 17
   tight, 16

Lamella, 146–8
Lamina, basal, 23–24, 184, 196–7
   dental, development of, 35–37, 42–43
   successional, 26, 42
   vestibular, 37, 42
Light microscopy, 1–4, (*Fig. 1.2*) 5
Lysosomes, 21

Malassez, epithelial cell rests of, 158–9, 164
Matrix vesicles, 78
Merism, 52–53
Mesenchyme, epithelial interaction with, 31–32
Mesial drift, 177–80
Mesodermal maintenance factor, 32
Microfilaments, 22
Microradiographic analysis of tissues, 9–10
Microtubules, 22
Microvilli, 18
Mineralization, 75–81, 97–99
Minerals in enamel, 126
Mitochondria, 21–22
Molar
   blood supply to, 64, (*Fig. 8.1*) 65
   clone, 44
   cusps, 49, 52, 53–54
   growth of, lower first deciduous, 57, (*Fig. 7.1*) 58
   upper primary, 57, (*Fig. 7.3*) 59
   height measurement, 60
   morphology, 46
Morphogenesis, 46–55
Mouth, embryonic development of, 35
Mucosa, oral, age changes in, 202
Myofibroblasts, 177

Nasmyth's membrane, 193–5
Nerve fibres, in dentine, 10, 109–12
   in periodontal ligament, 167–8
   in pulp, 200
Nerves, tooth bud development and, 37–38

INDEX

Neural crest, 28–30
  interactions, 33
Nucleus, cell, 18

Occlusal force, anterior component of, 178–9
Odontoblasts, development of, 30, 94–100, 158
  extent within dentinal tubules, 105–7
  function, 26, 105
  repair, 108
  transmission of stimulus by, 112–13
Organ, dental, 40
  growth of, 61
Organelles, ultrastructure of, (*Fig. 2.1*) 13
Osteogenesis, (*Fig. 10.7*) 84
Osteon, 90–91
Osteonectin, 78–79
Oxytalan fibres, 165–6

Pain, diffuseness of response to, 115
Papilla, dental, 26, 40, 48
  blood supply to, 65, (*Fig. 8.2*) 66
  growth of, 61, 156, 163
Pellicles, 197
Perikymata, 144–6
Periodontal ligament, age changes in, 201–2
  blood supply to, 66–67
  cells, 164
  collagen turnover in, 6–7, 72, 164, 167
  development, 39, 161–4
  effect on tooth movement, 174–7
  effect of width variation of, 153
  fibres, 164–5
  sensory function, 167–8
  structure, 164–5
  supportive function, 165–7
Periodontium, 161–8
Peroxisomes, 21
Phagocytosis, 15
Phase contrast microscopy, 3–4
Phospholipids, 15–16
Phosphoprotein, 78
Pinocytosis, 15
Plasma membrane 12–18
Preameloblast, (*Fig. 15.2*) 119
Precement, 150, 155
Preodontoblast, 48
Prism, cross striations, 141
  directions, 138–41

Prism, cross striations (*cont.*)
  formation, 126–35
  sheath, 141–4
  structure, 137–44
Procollagen, 70
Proline as radioactive marker, 6–7
Protein, analysis of, 8–9
  in ameloblast, 122–3
  in plasma membrane, 14
  shape determination of, 46
  synthesis, 19–20
Pseudopodium, 18
Pulp, age changes in, 200–1
  calcification, 201
  canal, 26–27
  stones, 201
Pulpo-periodontal canals, 156, 157, (*Fig. 18.2*) 158

Radioactive marker technique, 6–7
Retzius, striae of, 3, 144–6
Ribosomes, 19–20
RNA, 18–20
Root, anatomical, 26
  blood supply to, 65, 157
  dentinogenesis, (*Fig. 12.2*) 96
  diaphragm, 156
  formation, 156–60, 173
  sheath, 150, 156–60, 164

Scanning electron microscopy, 5–6
Scleroblast, 33
Section preparation, for electron microscopy, 4
  for light microscopy, 1–2
Sharpey's fibres, 27, 150, (*Fig. 17.1*) 151, 152
Silver staining, 2
Soft tissue *see under* Tissue
Spindles, 146–8
Staining for light microscopy, 1–2
Stellate cells, 18
Stellate reticulum, 40–41, 42, (*Fig. 15.1*) 118, 120–1
Stratum intermedium, 42, 121
Striae of Retzius, 3, 144–6

Terminal bar, 17, 121
Terminal web, 17

INDEX

Tissue, control of, 49–50
  hard, formation features of, (*Fig. 10.1*) 76
  genesis of, 75–88
  investigation of, 1–11
  soft, pressure causing tooth movement from, 179
Tomes granular layer, 26, 107–8
Tomes process, (*Fig. 15.3*) 120, 126–8, 132–4
Tooth, as age indicator, 202
  blood supply to, 63–67, 165–6, 174
  buds, 37–39, 40
  development, (*Fig. 3.1*) 25, 35–45, (*Fig. 18.3*) 159, 186
  embryonic, (*Fig. 5.2*) 36
  eruption, 172–7, 186
  follicle, 39, 40
  formation and induction, 28–33
  germ growth, 56–61, 161–2, 171–2
  height measurement, 58–60
  in situ, 25–27

Tooth, as age indicator (*cont.*)
  morphogenesis, 46–55
  movement, 153, 166–7, 171–80
  repair, 163
  sequence of development of, 43–44
  support, 165–7
Transmission electron microscopy, 4–5
Trans-septal fibre system, 166–7
  contraction of, 179
Tubules *see under* Dentine
Tufts, 146–8

Vascular network analysis, 63–64
Vitamin C deficiency, effect on collagen formation, 72, 167, 176
von Korff fibres, 96–97, (*Fig. 12.4*) 98

X-ray analysis of tissues, 9–10

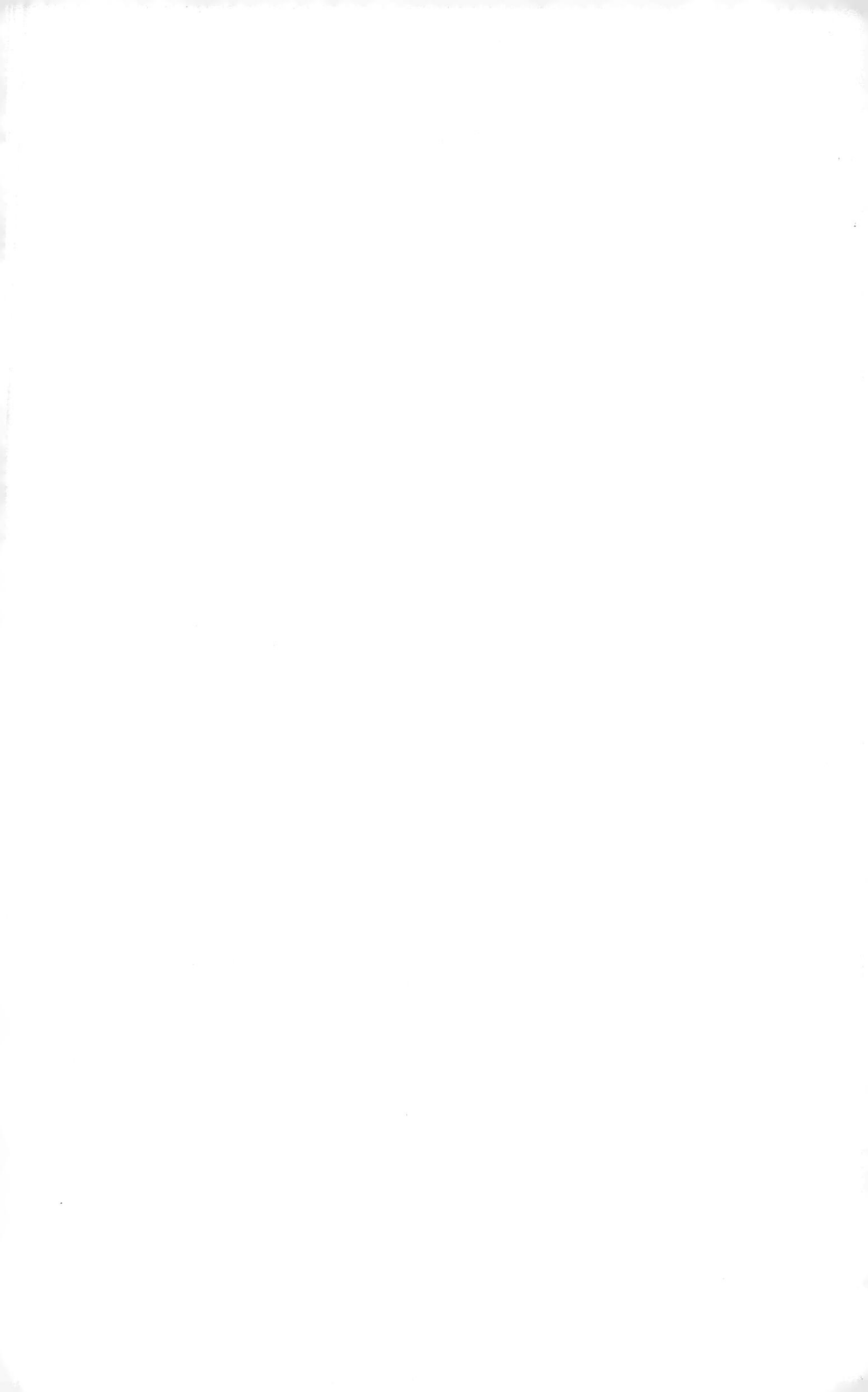